Carolina Marotta Ribeiro

Clinical and pathological aspects associated with otitis externa in dogs

Carolina Marotta Ribeiro

Clinical and pathological aspects associated with otitis externa in dogs

Evaluation of antimicrobial sensitivity in vitro and efficacy in vivo

ScienciaScripts

Imprint

Any brand names and product names mentioned in this book are subject to trademark, brand or patent protection and are trademarks or registered trademarks of their respective holders. The use of brand names, product names, common names, trade names, product descriptions etc. even without a particular marking in this work is in no way to be construed to mean that such names may be regarded as unrestricted in respect of trademark and brand protection legislation and could thus be used by anyone.

Cover image: www.ingimage.com

This book is a translation from the original published under ISBN 978-620-2-17522-7.

Publisher:
Sciencia Scripts
is a trademark of
Dodo Books Indian Ocean Ltd. and OmniScriptum S.R.L publishing group

120 High Road, East Finchley, London, N2 9ED, United Kingdom
Str. Armeneasca 28/1, office 1, Chisinau MD-2012, Republic of Moldova, Europe
Printed at: see last page
ISBN: 978-620-7-33429-2

Table of contents:

DEDICATORY

I dedicate this work to my Mother, wise and sovereign, who not only gave me life,
but teaches me how to live...

ACKNOWLEDGMENTS

This dissertation was only possible because of the valued friends and indispensable companions, whom I now thank.

To my advisor **Prof. Argemiro Sanavria** (Department of Epidemiology and Public Health) for his extreme patience in sharing his vast experience with a student who still has so much to learn. I am sincerely grateful to him for having remained a confident and present advisor at every stage of this dissertation. Your encouragement and companionship at all times, sharing valuable links from the most pleasant moments to the most difficult, makes me recognize you as a true friend as well as an advisor.

To my co-supervisor **Prof. Paulo Oldemar Scherer** (Department of Animal Biology) for his experience that was always sharing and for his competence that was always enthusiastic. I am especially grateful to him for having remained overly critical and essentially confident, for his always pertinent character in adding important aspects and for his proselytizing and friendly manner.

Prof. Angela de Oliveira and **Prof. Sergio Gaspar do Campos** (Department of Veterinary Microbiology and Immunology) for their ever-patient willingness to teach all the subjects I asked about and for the enjoyable Microbiology classes, which were essential for the composition of this dissertation. Thank you for your kindness in sharing so much experience.

To **Prof. Marcelo Abidu Figueiredo** (Department of Animal Biology) for his fundamental, essential and indispensable help with statistics, invaluable patience, prompt attention and vast competence in teaching and clarifying the most diverse doubts.

To the friends and colleagues from the Parasitic Diseases Laboratory who participated more directly in this dissertation, **Patrícia Giupponi Cardoso, Claúdia Bezerra da Silva, Joice Aparecida Rezende Vilena, Marcos Sandes Pires, Luíz Carlos Ribeiro da Paz and Cléa Guimaraes,** for their always enlightening discussions and their unceasing help at every stage of this dissertation. I am grateful for the friendship and advice of these brothers of mine, who were always eager to help and pertinent when adding.

To the DESP family, **Kelli Souza Melo, Dione Cristian Marques Silva, Marli Viana Pinheiro,**

Otacilho José Domingos, Cezar da Costa Generoso, Marta Elisabete da Silva, Ivana do Socorro Glins, Josemar Cezar Goncalves for the logistics, incessant affection, unrestricted and cosmopolitan support of the companions with whom I lived sweet and priceless moments of my existence.

To Mr. **Ataide Baptista** for his warm and contagious morning greetings.

To all the professors who have contributed so much to my personal and professional development in the Department of Epidemiology and Public Health and the Postgraduate Program in Veterinary Medicine.

Lorena Florencio de Oliveira and **Regina Helena de Oliveira Santos**, employees of the Veterinary Medicine Postgraduate Coordination Office, for being solicitous and competent, always present for the most important matters.

To the total and unrestricted support of my family, always willing to help me in everything. I would like to thank my mother, **Maria Marotta**, who was unconditional in all her actions, my brothers, **Humberto Marotta** and **Rodrigo Marotta**, for their essential and endless emotional and constructive support, and my animals *Taz* and *Frodo* for their inspiration and affection.

Most of all, I thank the good **GOD** and **Our Lady of Fátima, to** whom I am devoted, for always keeping me close and enlightening my life.

BIOGRAPHY

Born in Rio de Janeiro in 1983, daughter of Maria Marotta, sister of Humberto Marotta and Rodrigo Marotta. Attended elementary school at Colégio Imaculada Conceicao in Botafogo, elementary school at Colégio Municipal Minas Gerais in Urca, and high school at Colégio Pedro II in Sao Cristovao. I entered the UFRRJ in 2002, graduating in Veterinary Medicine in 2007. In 2009, I started a postgraduate course in Veterinary Medicine at UFRRJ.

EPIGRAPH

"When man learns to respect even the smallest creature, be it animal or plant, no one will need to teach him to love his fellow man"

Albert Shweitzer (Nobel Peace Prize winner, 1952).

SUMMARY

Otitis externa is the most common disease of the ear canal in dogs. This disease is painful, causes extreme discomfort and requires immediate treatment. The aim of this study was to describe the clinical and pathological aspects of otitis externa in naturally affected domestic dogs and to assess the in *vitro* sensitivity or *in vivo* clinical efficacy of the main antimicrobials used to treat this disease. Thirty-six animals took part in the study, totaling 72 ear *swab* samples of ear secretions collected from animals with clinical signs of otitis. Of the samples analyzed, 67 (93.1%) resulted in microbial growth, while 50 (69.4%) showed yeast growth. Among the 101 strains isolated were *Pseudomonas sp* 27 (26.7%), *Streptococcussp* 14 (13.9%) *Escherichia coli* 13 (12.9%), *Corynebacterium sp* 11 (10.9%), *Staphylococcus intermedius 10* (9.9%), *Staphylococcus* coagulase negative 10 (9.9%), *Staphylococcus aureus* 8 (7.9%), *Proteus sp* 4 (4%), *Bacillus sp 4 (4%)*. Pathological changes included erythema in 30 ears (41.7%), punctate hemorrhages in 48 (66.7%), erosions in 54 (75%), hyperemia in 62 (86.1%), edema in 52 (72.2%), thickening of the skin in 66 (91.7%), hyperpigmentation in 20 (27.8%), cartilage calcification 28 (38.9%), periauricular abrasions 52 (72.2%), partial stenosis 22 (30.5%), brown exudate 19 (26.3%), dark brown exudate 32 (44.4%), yellow exudate 24 (33.3%), intense exudate 50 (69.4%), moderate exudate 20 (27.8%), otohematoma eight (11.1%), pruritus 32 (88.9%), altered odor 36 (100%), hyperthermia nine (25%), hypocolored mucous membranes three (8.3%), mild dehydration three (8.3%), inappetence nine (25%), pre-parotid lymph node enlargement nine (25%), mandibular lymph node enlargement five (13.9%), otalgia 12 (33.3%), altered ear position five (13.9%), ear agitation 32 (88.9%) and head tilt four (11.1%). The antibiogram testing 17 antimicrobials indicated a treatment efficiency of over 70% for Chloramphenicol, Ciprofloxacin, Enrofloxacin, Gentamicin, Neomycin or Tobramycin. The percentage of cure using gentamicin, neomycin, enrofloxacin and/or ciprofloxacin reached 92%. In conclusion, gentamicin, neomycin and enrofloxacin showed better clinical efficiency in the treatment of canine otitis externa.

KEYWORDS: otitis externa, dog, bacteria, antibiogram and *in vivo* efficacy.

Chapter 1

1 INTRODUCTION

In Veterinary Medicine, most studies on canine otitis externa focus on the microbial isolation profile and the antimicrobial susceptibility of the isolated agents. More studies are needed that emphasize the importance of individualized clinical-pathological and laboratory evaluation associated with the etiology in cases of canine otitis externa, with a view to choosing the appropriate therapeutic protocol for successful treatment.

Otitis externa is the most common disease of the ear canal in dogs. This disease is painful, causes extreme discomfort and requires immediate treatment. Negligence in the treatment and management of animals can lead to chronic otitis and/or otitis media, which can result in impairment of the vestibulo-cochlear apparatus and rupture of the tympanic membrane, leading to loss of hearing and quality of life.

Irregular use and underdosing of otological products, especially when more than one active ingredient is combined, and without clinical and laboratory investigation, can lead to bacterial resistance and chronic infection.

The aim of this study is to describe the clinical-pathological aspects of otitis externa in naturally affected domestic dogs and to evaluate their sensitivity in *vitro and* clinical efficacy *in vivo, in* order to provide useful information for the development and application of diagnostic measures, effective treatments, prevention and control, thus guaranteeing hearing health and animal welfare.

Chapter 2

2 LITERATURE REVIEW

2.1. General aspects

Otitis externa is defined as inflammation of the ear canals and can involve the most proximal portion of the pinna (ROSYCHUK AND LUTTGEN, 2004). Otitis externa is no longer seen as an isolated disease of the ear canal, but rather as a syndrome that often reflects a systemic dermatological disease (JACOBSON, 2002). Otitis externa is the most commonly diagnosed disorder in dogs (GINEL, et al,2002).

Otitis represents around 8% to 15% of the cases of dogs referred for veterinary clinical assessment in Brazil (LEITE, 2000). It is estimated that otitis externa affects between 5% and 20% of dogs and 2% to 6% of cats and the incidence of tympanic perforation associated with otitis externa and otitis media is between 0.03% and 50% of cases (ROSYCHUK AND LUTTGEN, 2004). According to Farias (2002), chronic otitis externa accounts for 76.7% of cases of otopathy in dogs.

The microbiota of the external ear of dogs is made up of gram-positive cocci, gram-positive rods and yeasts of the *Malassezia pachydermatis* species (BONATES, 2003).

Otitis media involves the tympanic membrane. The tympanic membrane may be thickened or partially or completely ruptured, which makes it possible to infect the tympanic cavity, which is located more internally (COLE et al., 1998).

Otitis interna comprises inflammation of the semicircular canals, causing balance disorders. It is believed that most cases of otitis interna occur as an expansion of otitis media, which in turn is an expansion of otitis externa (HARVEY et al., 2004).

2.2. Anatomy of the Canine Ear

The ear is subdivided into the outer, middle and inner ear (HEINE, 2004). The auditory canal extends from the entrance of the vertical canal to the tympanic membrane.
The skin lining the canals consists of stratified squamous epithelium, sebaceous glands and ceruminous glands (modified apocrine glands). The sebaceous glands are found superficially in the dermis, while the ceruminous glands have a deeper distribution. A combination of ceruminous and sebaceous secretions in association with desquamated epithelium make up the normal cerumen that lines the auricular epithelium. The epidermis and dermis tend to become thinner as they progress towards the tympanic membrane, while the number of hair follicles and the amount of glandular tissue gradually decrease along the entire length of the canals (ROSYCHUK and LUTTGEN,

2004).

The external ear is made up of the outer and inner surfaces of the pinna and the vertical and horizontal auditory meatus. The pinna is lined on both sides by skin tissue which is strongly adhered to the periochondrial tissue. The ear canals are supported by the auricular and annular cartilages and, depending on the breed, can be five to 10 mm in diameter and up to two centimeters long at the canal. Their function is to receive air vibrations and conduct them to the tympanic membrane (HEINE, 2004).

The middle ear is lined by a mucous membrane made up of two layers of ciliated columnar epithelium, and is formed by the tympanic cavity and its walls, the medial surface of the tympanic membrane, the ossicles and their ligaments, muscles, nerves and the eustachian tube, which opens into the nasopharynx from the pharyngeal ostium of the auditory tube. The tympanic membrane is a thin, translucent, elliptical epithelial structure that separates the outer ear from the middle ear. The tympanic cavity is divided into three parts: dorsal, middle and ventral. Near or along the middle ear are branches of the facial and vagus nerves, and the carotid and lingual arteries (KUMAR and ROMAN-AUERHAHN, 2000).

The inner ear is formed by the cochlea, the semi-circular canals and the vestibular saccules (saccule and utricle), and is inserted into the petrous part of the temporal bone (HEINE, 2004).

2.3. Predisposing Factors

Factors such as temperature, humidity, anatomical predisposition and obstructive diseases of the ear canal are those that make the ear susceptible to inflammation of the ear canal due to primary factors (ROSYCHUK AND LUTTGEN, 2004).

The Cocker spaniel and the black Labrador have been shown to have relatively increased amounts of ceruminous glandular tissue, which may play a role in their predisposition to otitis externa (ROSYCHUK and LUTTGEN, 2004).

According to Gotthelf (2000), some conditions found in the ear canal favor the development of otitis externa, including stenosis, excess hair and cerumen, trauma and obstruction by tumors or polyps in the ear canal.

2.4. Primary Factors

The primary factors of otitis externa are those capable of initiating inflammation, hypersensitivity disorders, atopic dermatitis, hypersensitivity to arthropod saliva, pharmacodermia, foreign bodies, ectoparasites, the most common being *Demodex canis, Sarcoptes scabiei, Otodectes cyrotis,* idiopathic otitis and autoimmune diseases (ROSYCHUK AND LUTTGEN, 2004).

2.5. Perpetuating Factors

These are responsible for the continuation of the inflammatory response, even though the original primary factors may no longer be present or active, such as bacterial and fungal colonization by *Malassezia sp.,* chronic progressive pathological changes, otitis media and treatment failure (ROSYCHUK AND LUTTGEN, 2004, GOTTHELF, 2000).

2.6. Pathogenesis and Clinical Signs

During the early stages of otitis externa, there are varying degrees of erythema in the auricle, external meatus and canal lining (ROSSER, 2004). Because the ear canal is surrounded by cartilage, edema causes constriction of the canal's internal lumen, causing compression and pain. Histologically, mild to moderate hyperkeratosis, vasodilation of the dermis and edema are observed. The sebaceous glands undergo hyperplasia in the early stages of acute otitis, resulting in excessive production of cerumen (STOUT-GRAHAM et al., 1990). As the inflammation progresses, there is mixed intradermal infiltration of lymphocytes, mast cells and polymorphonuclear cells. The epithelia of the ear canal and tympanic membrane continue to increase in thickness, due to acanthosis and hyperkeratosis. Once otitis becomes chronic, the apocrine (ceruminous) glands begin to enlarge significantly, becoming hyperproductive. Therefore, an important perpetuating factor in chronic otitis is the progressive proliferation of the epidermis and dermis of the ear canal (ANGUS et al., 2002). In this case, when previous inflammation is not successfully treated, proliferation of the epithelial lining, sebaceous glands and ceruminous glands of the ear canal will occur, followed later by fibrosis and calcification of the cartilage (LOGAS, 1994).

The main symptoms observed in otitis externa during direct inspection are erythema, edema, scaling, ear alopecia, drooping of the head, itching, ulceration, pain, otohematoma and exudate (SCOTT, 2001).

Blackish exudate is usually associated with the presence of otoacariasis. *Staphylococcus sp.* infections usually produce a brownish or yellowish exudate. *Pseudomonas aeruginosa* and *Proteus sp.* infections are usually associated with a slightly yellowish, copious and fetid purulent exudate. Infections perpetuated by *Malassezia pachydermatis* present a chocolate brown ceruminous exudate (GOTTHELF, 2004).

2.7. Diagnosis

In cases of otitis externa, a systematic assessment of the patient is necessary through clinical history, anamnesis, general clinical examination, otoscopy, cytology, culture and antibiogram, as well as biopsy in otitis media and in recurrent and severe cases (JACOBSON, 2002). Culture and antibiograms should also be recommended in cases of chronic or recurrent otitis media (SCOTT et al, 2001, MALAYERI, 2010). According to Penna et al. (2009) after studying the antimicrobial resistance of isolates from 151 dogs with a clinical diagnosis of otitis, they concluded that the results show the recognition and potential need for bacterial culture with species identification and antimicrobial sensitivity tests for appropriate antimicrobial therapy.

A detailed dermatological history and complete physical examination should be carried out on all pets with ear disease. Examination of the ear should include assessment of the concave and convex surfaces of the pinna and palpation of the ear cartilages in the canals for pain, thickening and/or calcification. (ROSYCHUK and LUTTGEN, 2004).

Otoscopic examination should include the observation of parasites, the degree of inflammation within the canals, the size of the canals, the quantity and nature of the exudate, proliferative changes and the appearance of the tympanic membrane (SCOTT et al, 2001; ROSYCHUK and LUTTGEN, 2004).

The following organisms can be identified in the cytological examination of ears with otitis externa: cocci (*Staphylococcus sp., Streptococcus sp.*), rods (*Pseudomonas sp., Proteus sp,* and other gram-negative bacteria), yeasts (*Malassezia sp. and Candida sp.*) (TATER et al, 2003).

The cytology of the external auditory canal is characterized by the presence of squamous cells, epithelial cells and low numbers of commensals and potentially pathogenic microorganisms (GINEL et al, 2002).

Video-otoscopy is an effective method for quickly and safely visualizing the external auditory canal. It is a useful procedure in the diagnosis and prognosis of ear disorders (MANISCALCO et al., 2009).

2.8. Therapeutics

The general goals of otitis externa therapy are to control or remove the primary factors, reduce inflammation, resolve bacterial or yeast infections, and clean and dry the ears. These goals are usually achieved through the appropriate use of topical and sometimes systemic therapies (ROSYCHUK and LUTTGEN, 2004).

Most topical medications indicated for the treatment of otitis externa contain glucocorticoids in combination with antifungals and/or antibiotics. These combination products work well because otitis externa, regardless of the primary cause, tends to involve similar pathological changes: in more acute cases, edema, hyperemia and thickening of the stratum corneum (hyperkeratosis); in more chronic cases, epidermal hyperplasia, inflammatory cell infiltrates, dilation and hyperplasia of the ceruminous glands and dermal fibrosis. Colonization and infection with bacteria and yeasts are common (SCOTT et al, 2001; ROSYCHUK and LUTTGEN, 2004).

The treatment of otitis with antimicrobials, especially those with heavy exudation (suggestive of intense bacterial proliferation), should be carried out for at least one epithelial cycle, i.e. around 21 days (LEITE, 2008).

Topical antibacterial agents are indicated when infection, whether primary or perpetuating, is present. Aminoglycosides, neomycin, polymyxin and gentamicin, are potent topical antibiotics with good activity against pathogens commonly found in otitis externa. Polymyxin B is inactivated by pus and should only be used in clean ears.

Gram-negative infections resistant to gentamicin can be successfully treated with injectable amikacin (50mg/mL), applied in doses of three and five drops in each ear canal every 12 hours. However, aminoglycosides can be ototoxic with prolonged use or when used in animals with ruptured eardrums (SCOTT et al, 2001; LEITE 2008).

Antifungal agents are necessary in any case complicated or caused by yeasts, generally responding well to topical 1% miconazole or clotrimazole. Povidone iodine or chlorhexidine are also effective (SCOTT et al, 2001; ROSYCHUK and LUTTGEN, 2004).

Parasiticidal agents are indicated in ear products for *Otodectosis,* less commonly for *Demodex.* Most cases respond to products containing permethrin. In addition to using an effective parasiticide, two important points should be considered. Many animals can be asymptomatic carriers of *Otodectes* and all contacting animals, both cats and dogs, should be treated. *Otodectes* can be found in other areas of the body. Therefore, the whole body needs to be treated with effective parasiticides. The *Otodectes* life cycle requires treatment of the ear and body and should continue for at least three weeks, with a month being necessary in some cases. Some vets recommend topical application of ivermectin (ear drops), especially in cats. Amitraz (1mL of amitraz in 29 mL of mineral oil) is also effective when applied as ear drops (SCOTT et al 2001; ROSYCHUK and LUTTGEN, 2004).

Systemic treatment is indicated in cases of severe, chronic otitis externa or if otitis media is present; when owners are unable to administer topical treatments and, in some cases, when marked proliferative changes are present. Appropriate antibiotics or antifungals should be used up to a week after clinical cure, which usually requires therapy for six to eight weeks (SCOTT et al, 2001; ROSYCHUK and LUTTGEN, 2004). According to Leite (2008), the main antibiotics used to combat gram-negative bacteria are polymyxin B, aminoglycosides (gentamicin, neomycin and tobramycin) and quinolones (enrofloxacin, orbifloxacin and difloxacin). Ivermectin is an extremely effective systemic treatment for *Otodectes* infection. Collies and their crossbreeds should not be treated with ivermectin (SCOTT et al, 2001; ROSYCHUK and LUTTGEN, 2004).

Chapter 3

3 MATERIAL AND METHODS

3.1. Period:

This study was carried out between January and November 2010.

3.2. Animals:

Thirty-six dogs of different breeds, ages, sexes and sizes took part in the study. Each animal was given a medical record with a registration number and summary data to facilitate identification.

3.3. Animal containment

The animals were placed on a table and physically restrained with their hands and muzzles.

3.4. Clinical Examination

The animals were subjected to direct clinical inspection using a veterinary otoscope (before and after ear cleaning to remove excess exudate) of the outer ear and pinna. Physical examination, assessing mucous membrane color, skin turgor, body temperature and history.

3.5. Study Location

Animals living in the municipality of Seropédica.

3.6. Clinical and laboratory monitoring of animals

The animals were monitored with the authorization and prior guidance of the owners, through a detailed general and specific clinical examination according to a pre-established protocol and the data recorded on individual forms containing data on reviews, management and macroscopic aspects of the external ear and right and left ear pinna, by direct clinical inspection (figure 01) and with the aid of a veterinary otoscope.

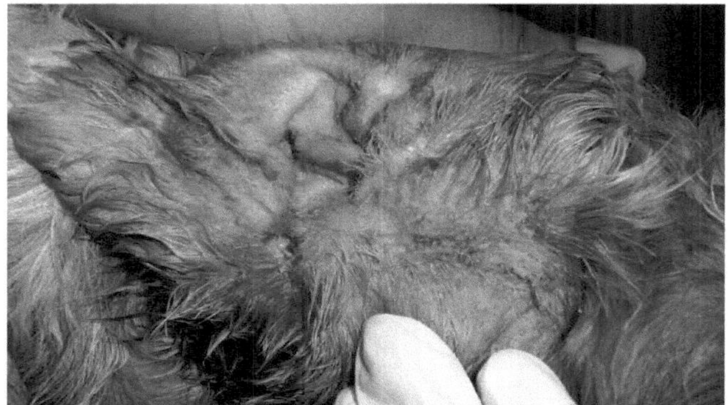

Figure 01 - Photomacrography: direct clinical inspection of the external ear of a Cocker spaniel canine with recurrent purulent otitis.

During the physical examination, the pre-parotid and mandibular lymph nodes were palpated, the color of the mucous membranes was assessed, as well as skin turgor, otalgia, changes in the position of the head and agitation of the ears, rectal temperature, the presence of appetite, behavioral changes and concomitant illnesses. Laboratory tests include aerobic bacterial culture and bilateral mycological culture of the outer ear.

The 72 samples of bilateral ear secretions were collected, without sedation, by inserting a dry sterile *swab* with *Stuart's* medium into the vertical portion of the external ear canal (figure 02), taking care not to contaminate it through contact with the external ear canal. The samples were immersed in culture medium, kept refrigerated and sent to the Parasitic Diseases Laboratory at the Federal Rural University of Rio de Janeiro within 24 hours of collection.

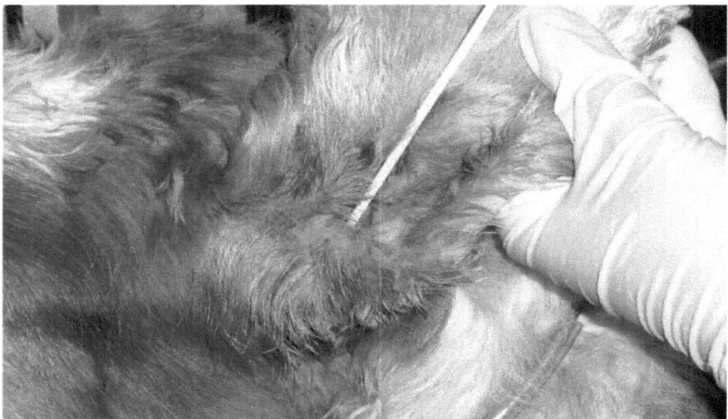

Figure 02- Photomacrography: collection of ear secretion samples by inserting a sterile *swab* into the vertical portion of the external auditory canal of a Cocker spaniel canine.

It was used from bacterial isolation to verify the presence and morphological study of microbial agents (bacterial and/or fungal) through Gram staining.

The bacteriological culture was carried out in the Parasitic Diseases Laboratory and the mycological culture was carried out in the Microbiology Laboratory of the Veterinary Institute of the UFRRJ. For the microbiological identification of the bacterial and yeast genus and/or species, the ear secretion samples were sown on 5% Sheep's Blood Agar, Chromagar Orientation (Figure 03) and Sabouraud Agar with Mycosel® . The Blood Agar plates were incubated in aerobiosis at 37° C for 24-72 hours (Figure 04). The chromogenic medium plates for the isolation and differentiation of pathogens were incubated at 37° C for 24-48 hours.

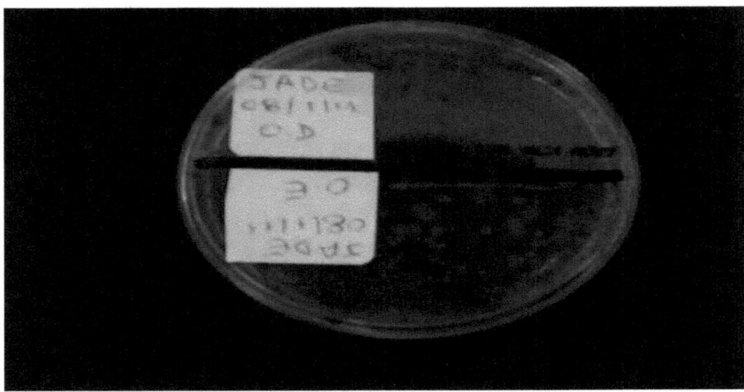

Figure 03- Photomacography: samples of auricular secretions sown in Chromagar Orientation Medium.

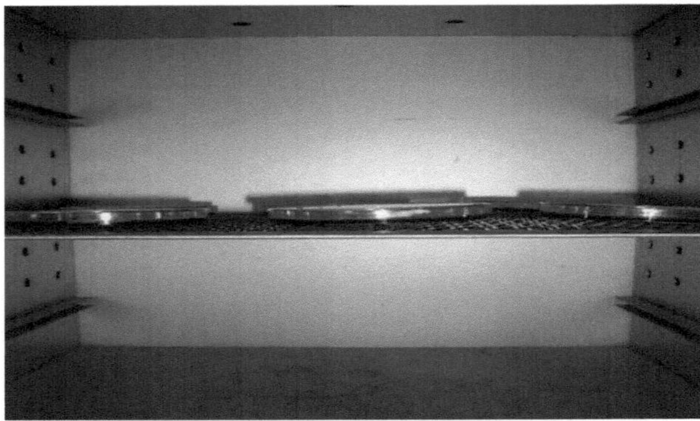

Figure 04- Photomacography: Blood Agar plates incubated in aerobiosis at 37 C.°

The samples were identified and classified according to Quinn et al, 2005. The Sabouraud agar plates were incubated in aerobiosis at 28° C for seven days.

If bacterial growth was absent in the direct plating, a second attempt at bacterial isolation was made using BHI brain infusion broth (Figure 05).

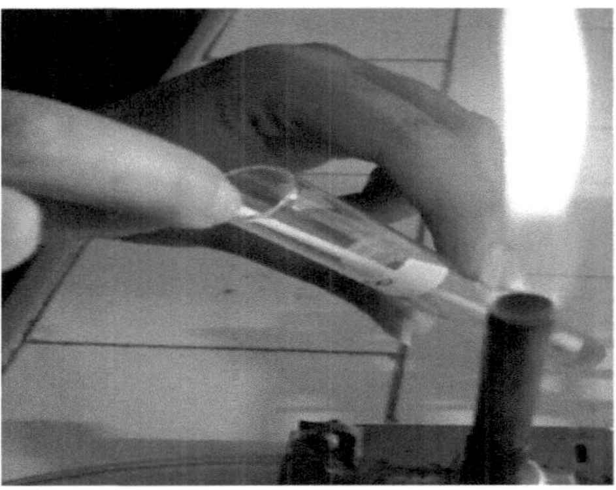

Figure 05- Photomacography: *Swabs,* with a sample of canine ear secretion, transferred to BHI broth.

The Sabouraud Agar plates were examined daily up to seven days after sowing in order to obtain colonies of *Malassezia pachydermatis* or any other yeast present.

The *swabs* containing the samples were transferred to BHI broth, incubated at 37^0 C and then sown in Petri dishes containing Muller Hinton Agar for the antibiogram containing the main antibiotics recommended for the treatment of canine otitis externa (figure 06). The standard antibiogram was carried out with a strain of *Staphylococcus aureus* (ATCC 6538P).

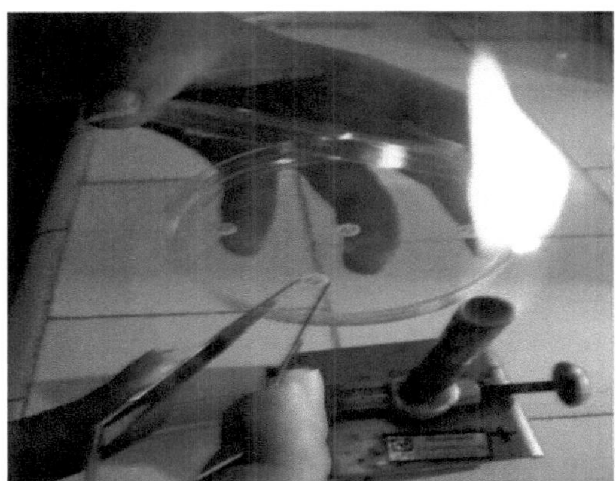

Figure 06 - Photomacography: *in vitro* desensitization tests, single disk diffusion method.

To *carry out the in vitro* sensitivity tests, the single disk diffusion method was used, testing 17 antimicrobials (Figure 07): _ Beta-lactams: penicillin (10 u.i.), ampicillin (10 µg), amoxicillin (10 µg), amoxicillin with clavulanic acid (20/10 µg), cephalothin (30 µg), cefoxitin (30 µg). _ Aminoglycosides: neomycin (30µg), gentamicin (10µg), tobramycin (10 µg) Macrolides:

azithromycin$^{(10\ \mu g)}$; _ Quinolones: enrofloxacin ciprofloxacin $^{(10\ \mu g),\ (5\ \mu g)}$; _ Other classes: tetracycline$^{(30\ \mu g)}$, chloramphenicol$^{(30\ \mu g)}$, sulfa with trimethoprim (25 µg), clidamycin$^{(2\ \mu g)}$, polymyxin B (300 u.i.).

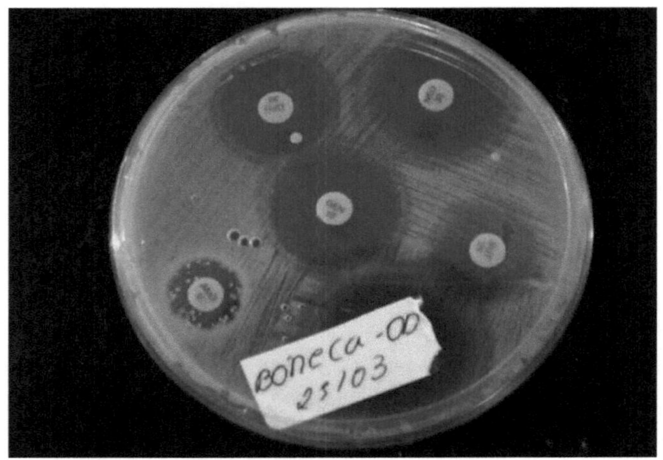

Figure 07- Photomacography: *in vitro* sensitivity tests, single disk diffusion method.

According to the results of the antibiogram, the owners were given therapeutic advice for the treatment of bacterial and mixed otitis media. The treatments consisted of topical antimicrobials, anti-inflammatories and antifungals, with or without systemic medication, applied every 12 hours for 21 days after removing the exudate/cerumen with ceruminol. Fourteen days after the end of treatment, samples of bilateral ear secretions were collected for bacteriological culture, otoscopy and direct clinical examination. Cure was confirmed when the animal was restored to clinical normality and there was no microbial growth or macroscopic lesions in the external ear.

Chapter 4

4. RESULTS AND DISCUSSION

4.1. Total number of ear secret samples analyzed:

Thirty-six animals took part in the study, totaling 72 samples of right and left ear *swabs* containing ear secretions collected from animals with clinical signs of otitis. Of these, 72 (100%) were submitted to bacteriological and mycological culture.

4.2. Microbiological growth of ear secretion samples submitted to bacterial and mycological culture

Of the 72 samples analyzed, 67 (93.1%) resulted in microbial growth, while 5 (6.9%) were negative, showing no growth of bacteria or yeasts, and were sterile to the culture used (graph 01).

Graph 01: Microbial growth of ear secretion samples.

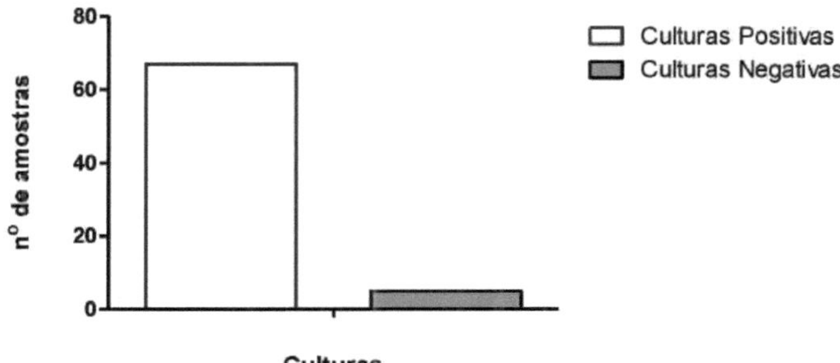

4.3. Microorganisms isolated among the positive samples submitted to bacterial and mycological culture:

Of the total of 67 positive samples, 38 (56.7%) showed an association between bacteria and yeast, while 17 (25.4%) resulted only in a bacterial culture and 12 (17.9%) in a single yeast culture (graph 02).

Graph 02: Microbiological isolation from ear secretion samples.

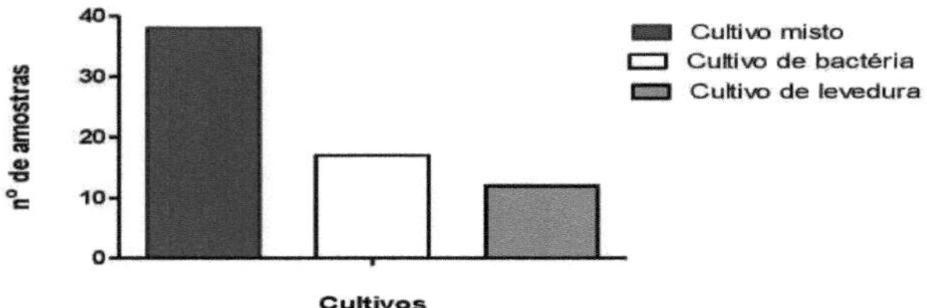

4.4. Total number of ear secretion samples submitted to bacterial culture:

Of the 72 samples analyzed, 55 (76.4%) showed bacterial growth, while 17 (23.6%) did not (graph 03).

Graph 03: Ear secretion samples submitted for bacterial cultivation.

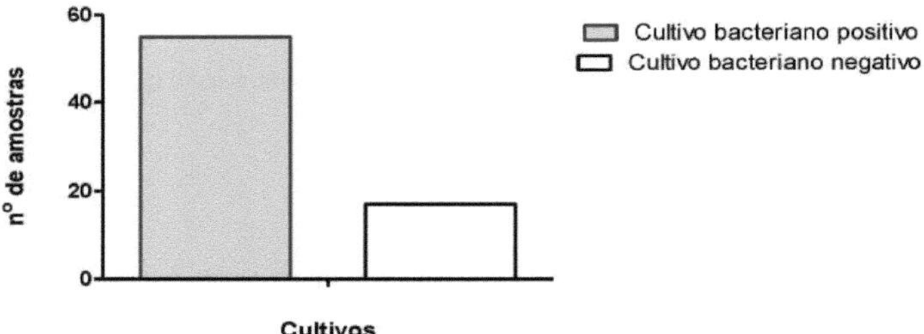

4.5. Total number of ear secretion samples submitted to mycological culture:

Of the 72 samples analyzed, 50 (69.4%) showed yeast growth, while 22 (30.1%) showed no growth (graph 04).

Graph 04: Canine ear secretion samples submitted to yeast culture.

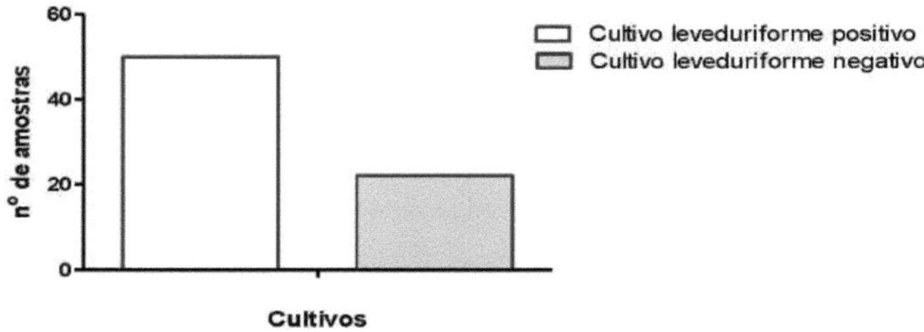

4.6. Prevalence of single and multiple bacterial infections in ear secretion samples:

From a total of 55 samples that resulted in positive bacterial cultures, 101 strains were obtained. Of these samples, 19 (34.5%) resulted in a single bacterial culture, yielding 19 strains. The isolation of two bacterial species from one sample occurred in 21 (38.2%) cultures, yielding 42 strains. Among the samples, 14 (25.4%) resulted in the isolation of three or more distinct species, yielding 43 strains (Graph 05).

Graph 05: Bacterial isolation of one or more bacteria:

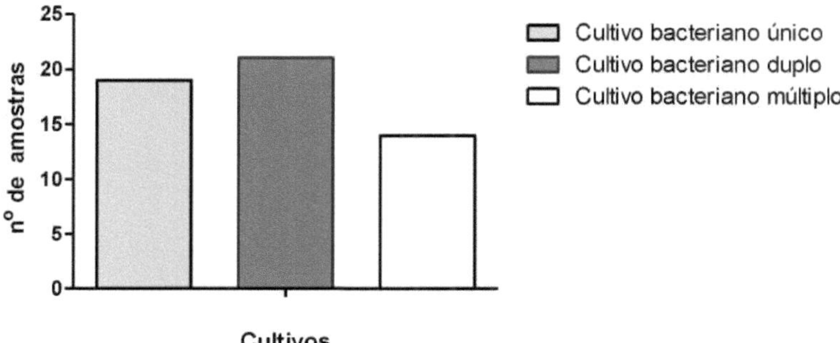

4.7. Gram-positive and gram-negative bacterial prevalence in ear secretion samples:

Among the 101 bacterial strains obtained, there were more gram-positive bacteria (57 cultures or 56.4%) than gram-negative bacteria (44 cultures or 43.6%), Graph 06.

Graph 06: Bacterial prevalence in terms of cell wall type.

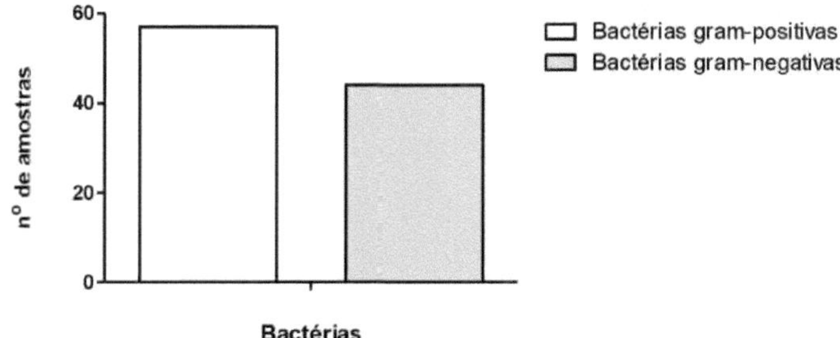

4.8. Bacterial prevalence in ear secretion samples:

Among the 101 strains isolated, the most prevalent species was *Pseudomonas sp* 27 (26.7%), followed by *Streptococcus sp* 14 (13.9%) *Escherichia coli* 13 (12.9%), *Corynebacterium sp* 11 (10.9%), Staphylococcus intermedius 10 (9.9%), Staphylococcus coagase negative 10 (9.9%), Staphylococcus aureus 8 (7.9%,9%), *Staphylococcus intermedius* 10 (9.9%), *Staphylococcus coagulase negative* 10 (9.9%), *Staphylococcus aureus* 8 (7.9%), *Proteus sp* 4 (4%), *Bacillus sp* 4 (4%), graph 07.

Graph 07: Bacterial prevalence in canine ear secretion samples.

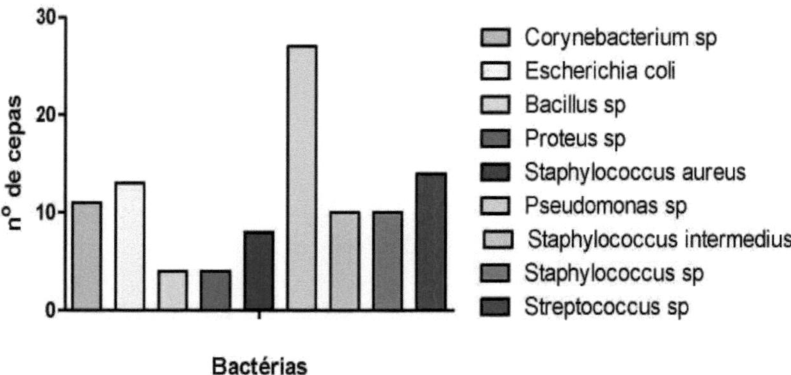

4.9. Yeast prevalence in canine ear secretion samples:

Of the 72 samples analyzed, the yeast species *Malassezia pachydermatis* was isolated in 50 cultures (69.4%), while in 22 cultures (30.6%) nothing was isolated (graph 08).

Graph 08: Yeast culture from ear-secretion samples.

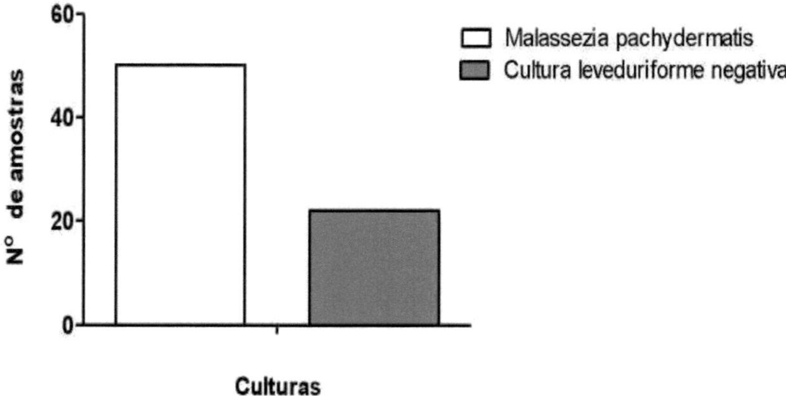

4.10. Specific bacterial prevalence in ear secretion samples that resulted in mixed bacterial culture:

From the ear samples that resulted in the growth of two or more different bacteria, it is possible to see variation in bacterial prevalence, as shown in Table 01.

Table 01: Bacteria isolated in single and multiple bacterial cultures:

Bacteria	Unique cultivation		Multiple cropping	
	Total	%	Total	%
Pseudomonas sp	1	5,3	26	32,9
Streptococcus sp	2	10,5	12	15,2
E. coli	0	0	13	16,5
Corynebacterium sp	7	36,8	4	5,1
S. intermedius	1	5,3	9	11,4
Staphylococcus sp	3	15,8	7	8,9
S. aureus	3	15,8	5	6,3
Proteus sp	0	0	4	5,1
Bacillus sp	2	10,5	2	2,5
Total	19	100	82	100

4.11. Bacterial associations observed in multiple bacterial infections:

Table 02 shows the bacterial associations that occurred when more than one bacterium was isolated from an ear *swab* sample.

Table 02: Specific bacterial associates found in multiple bacterial infections:

Bacterial associates	Total	%
Streptococcus sp and *Pseudomonas sp*	4	5,6
Pseudomonas sp, E. coli and *S. intermedius*	4	5,6
Pseudomonas sp and *S. intermedius*	3	4,2
Streptococcus sp, Pseudomonas sp and *E. coli*	3	4,2
Pseudomonas sp, E. coli and *Staphylococcus sp*	2	2,8
Streptococcus sp, Pseudomonas sp and *S. aureus*	2	2,8
Streptococcus sp and *E. coli*	2	2,8
Proteus sp and *S. aureus*	2	2,8
Pseudomonas sp and *Corynebacterium sp*	2	2,8
Pseudomonas sp and *Staphylococcus sp*	2	2,8
Proteus sp and *Bacillus sp*	1	1,4

Proteus sp and *Corynebacterium sp*	1	1,4
Pseudomonas sp and *E. coli*	1	1,4
Streptococcus sp, *Pseudomonas sp* and *S. intermedius*	1	1,4
Staphylococcus sp and *E. coli*	1	1,4
Pseudomonas sp and *S. aureus*	1	1,4
Pseudomonas sp, *S. aureus* and *Staphylococcus sp*	1	1,4
Pseudomonas sp, *E. coli*, *Corynebacterium sp* and *Bacillus sp*	1	1,4
Total multiple crops	34	47,2

4.12. Association between bacteria and yeasts observed in mixed infections:

Table 03 shows the associations between yeasts and bacteria.

Table 03: Association between yeasts and bacteria obtained:

Bacterial associates	Total	%
Proteus sp, *Bacillus sp* and *Malassezia pachydermatis*	2	2,8

Pseudomonas sp, E. coli, S.intermedius and Malassezia pachydermatis	2	2,8
Proteus sp, S. aureus and Malassezia pachydermatis	2	2,8
Corynebacterium sp and Malassezia pachydermatis	7	9,7
Staphylococcus sp and Malassezia pachydermatis	4	5,6
Staphylococcus sp, E. coli and Malassezia pachydermatis	1	1,4
Streptococcus sp and Malassezia pachydermatis	1	1,4
S. aureus and Malassezia pachydermatis	1	1,4
Streptococcus sp, Pseudomonas sp and Malassezia pachydermatis	5	6,9
Corynebacterium sp, E. coli, Pseudomonas sp, Bacillus sp and Malassezia pachydermatis	1	1,4
Bacillus sp and Malassezia pachydermatis	2	2,8
Staphylococcus sp, Pseudomonas sp and Malassezia pachydermatis	2	2,8

S.intermedius and Malassezia pachydermatis	1	1,4
Streptococcus sp , E. coli, S.intermedius and Malassezia pachydermatis	1	1,4
Pseudomonas sp, E. coli and Malassezia pachydermatis	1	1,4
Pseudomonas sp, and Malassezia pachydermatis	1	1,4
Pseudomonas sp, E. coli, Staphylococcus sp and Malassezia pachydermatis	2	2,8
Streptococcus sp, E. coli and Malassezia pachydermatis	2	2,8
Total bacterial cultures associated with yeast	38	52,8

4.13. Distribution of samples by gender:

Of the 36 animals that took part in the study, 19 (52.8%) were males and 17 (47.2%) were females, showing a predominance of males with otitis.

There was no statistically significant difference (P>0.05) between bacterial and non-bacterial otitis. There was a statistically significant difference (P<0.05) in gender between fungal and non-fungal otitis media (graph 09). There was no statistically significant difference (P>0.05) as to gender between mixed and non-mixed otitis media.

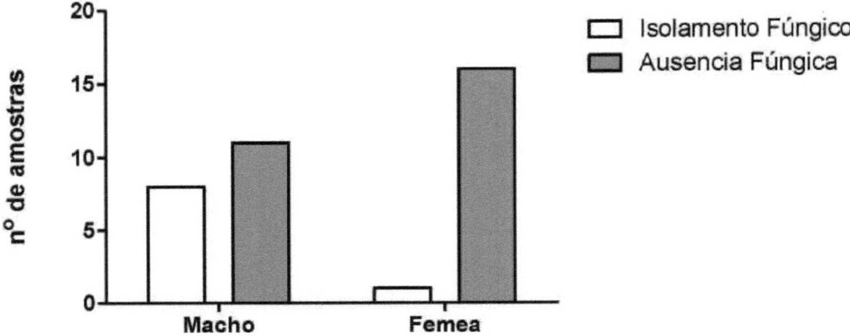

Graph 09: Distribution of samples according to sex and fungal isolation:

4.14. Distribution of samples according to age group:

Of the 36 animals, two (5.6%) belonged to group "A" (animals up to one year old), 20 (55.6%) belonged to group "B" (over one to five years old), 15 (41.7%) belonged to group "C" (over five to ten years old) and three (8.3%) belonged to group "D" (over ten years old), as shown in graph 11. A lower prevalence of otitis was observed in animals up to one year old, belonging to group "A", and in animals over ten years old, belonging to group "D". It was observed that the animals in groups "B" (over one year old up to five years old) and "C" (over five to ten years old) had a higher number of cases of otitis (graph 10). There was no statistical difference between the groups (p > 0.05).

Graph 10: Distribution of animals by age group.

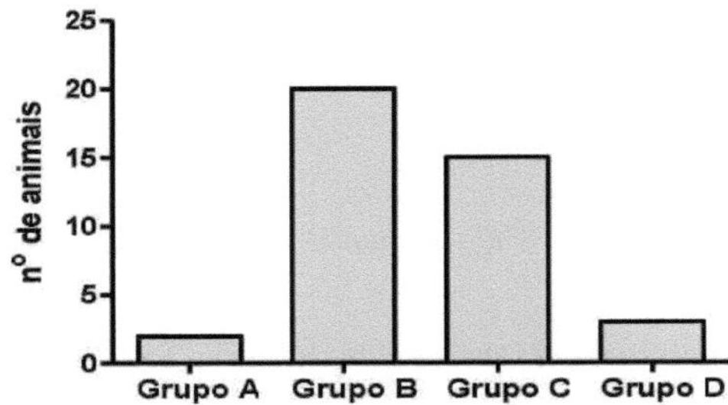

4.15. Distribution of animals by breed:

Among the 36 animals studied, the canine breeds observed were eight (22.2%) Poodles, seven (19.4%) Labrador retrivier seven (19.4%) SRD (no defined breed), three (8,3%) Cockers spaniel, two (5.6%) Beagles, two (5.6%) Shitzus, two (5.6%) Chowchows, two (5.6%) Pitbulls, one (2.8%) Boxer, one (2.8%) German Shepherd, one (2.8%) Dalmatian (graph 11). Among the animals that took part in the study, there was a higher frequency of the Poodle breed, Labrador retrivier and those with no defined breed.

Graph 11: Distribution of animals by breed.

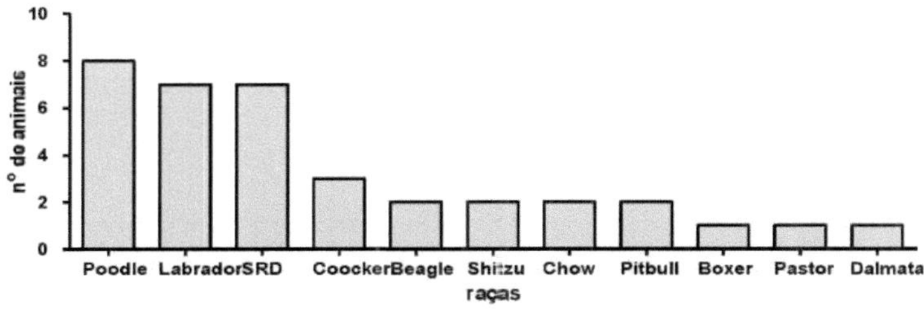

Table 04: Distribution of animals by breed.

Ra?a	Number of animals	%
Poodle	8	22,2
SRD	7	19,4
Labrador retriver	7	19,4
Cocker spaniel	3	8,3
Chowchow	2	5,6
Beagle	2	5,6
Shitzu	2	5,6
Pitbull	2	5,6

Dalmatian	1	2,8
German Shepherd	1	2,8
Boxer	1	2,8
Total	36	100

4.16. Distribution of otitis samples according to animal size:

Of the 36 animals, eight (22.2%) were small, 14 (38.9%) medium-sized and 14 (38.9%) large. Most of the animals studied were medium or large, but there was no statistical difference between them in terms of bacterial, fungal and mixed otitis media.

Table 05: Distribution of bacterial otitis samples according to animal size.

Size	Bacterial isolation	%
Small	3	33,3
Medium	3	33,3
Large	3	33,3
Total	9	100
(p < 0,05).		

Table 06: Distribution of fungal otitis samples according to size of the animal.

Size	Fungal isolation	%
Small	0	0
Medium	5	55,5
Large	4	44,4
Total	9	100
(p < 0,05).		

Table 07: Distribution of mixed otitis samples according to animal size.

Size	Mixed Insulation	%
Small	4	25
Medium	5	31,2
Large	7	43,7
Total	16	100
(p < 0,05).		

4.17. Distribution of otitis samples according to ear morphology:

Of the 36 animals, 18 (50%) had pendulous ears, 15 (41.7%) had semi-pendulous ears and three (8.3%) had erect ears (graph 12). Most of the animals had pendulous ears.

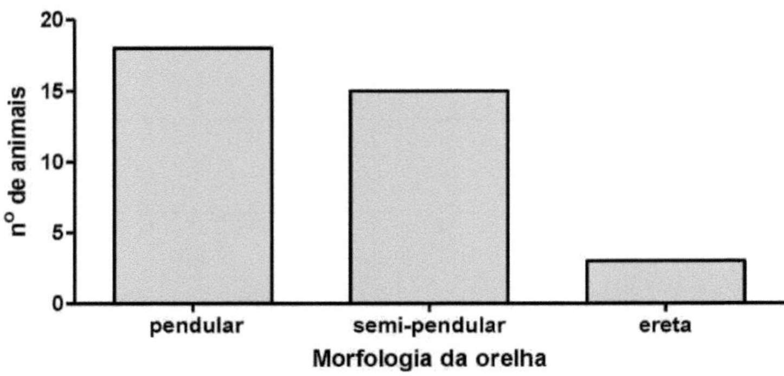

Graph 12: Distribution of ear secretion samples according to ear morphology.

As for bacterial and non-bacterial otitis, there was no statistically significant difference (p > 0.05) between ear morphology (table 08).

Table 08: Distribution of bacterial otitis samples according to ear morphology.

Ear morphology	Bacterial isolation	%
Pendular	6	66,6
Semi-pendicular	2	22,2
Ereta	1	11,1
Total	9	100
(p > 0,05).		

As for fungal and non-fungal otitis, there was a statistically significant difference (p < 0.05) between ear morphology (Table 09).

Table 09: Distribution of fungal otitis samples according to ear morphology.

Ear morphology	Fungal isolation	%
Pendular	6	66,6

Semi-pendicular	3	33,3
Ereta	0	0
Total	9	100
(p < 0,05).		

As for mixed and non-mixed otitis, there was no statistically significant difference (p > 0.05) between ear morphology (Table 10).

Table 10: Distribution of mixed otitis samples according to ear morphology.

Ear morphology	Mixed Insulation	%
Pendular	5	31,2
Semi-pendicular	10	62,5
Ereta	1	6,2
Total	16	100
(p > 0,05).		

4.18. Distribution of otitis samples according to the animal's coat:

Of the 36 animals, 16 (44.4%) had short coats, 15 (41.7%) had medium coats and five (13.9%) had long coats (graph 13). Most cf the animals had short coats.

Graph 13: Distribution of ear secret_on samples according to the animal's coat.

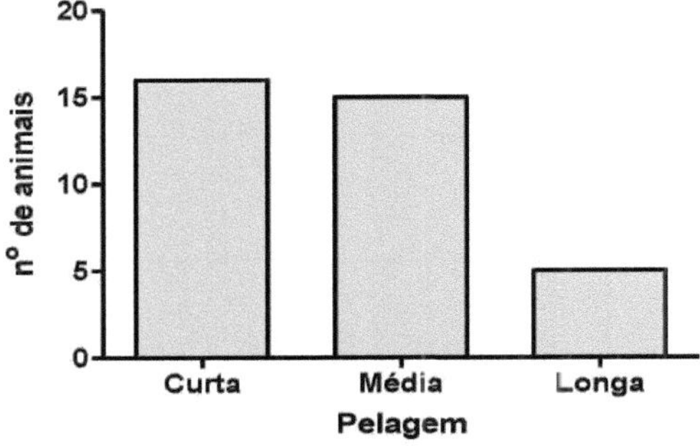

With regard to bacterial and mixed otitis, there was a statistically significant difference (p <0.05) between the animals of different coats. For fungal otitis, there was no statistical difference.

Table 11: Distribution of bacterial otitis samples according to the animal's coat.

Type of coat	Bacterial isolation	%
Short	1	11,1
Media	4	44,4
Long	4	44,4
Total	9	100
(p <0,05).		

Table 12: Distribution of fungal otitis samples according to the animal's coat type.

Type of coat	Fungal isolation	%
Short	4	44,4
Media	4	44,4
Long	1	44,4
Total	9	100
(p >0,05)		

Type of coat	Mixed Insulation	%
Short	11	68,7
Media	5	31,2
Long	0	0
Total	16	100
*p > 0,05).		

4.19. Distribution of otitis samples according to ear size:

Of the 36 animals, two (5.6%) had small ears, 12 (33.3%) had medium ears and 12 (33.3%) had large ears (graph 14). Most of the animals studied had medium and large ears.

Graph 14: Distribution of ear secretion samples according to ear size.

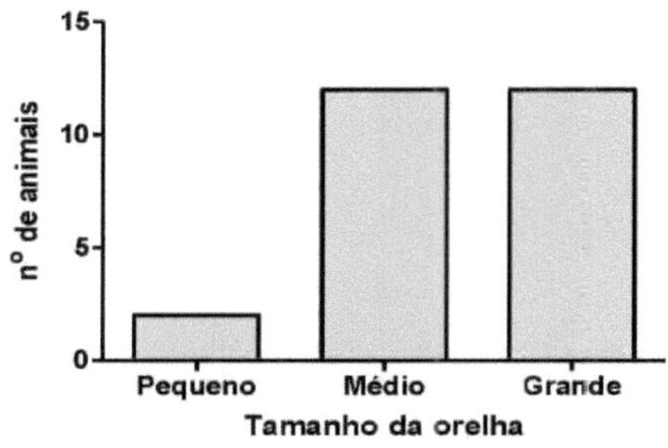

As for bacterial and non-bacterial otitis, there was a statistically significant difference (p <

0.05) between ear size (Table 14).

Table 14: Distribution of bacterial otitis samples according to the size of the animal's ear.

Ear size	Bacterial isolation	%
Small	2	22,2
Average	7	77,8
Large	0	0
Total	9	100
(p < 0,05).		

As for fungal and non-fungal otitis, there was no statistically significant difference (p > 0.05) between ear sizes (Table 15).

Table 15: Distribution of fungal otitis auricular secretion samples according to the size of the animal's ear.

Ear size	Fungal isolation	%
Small	0	0
Average	6	66,7

Large	3	33,3
Total	9	100
(p > 0,05).		

As for mixed and non-mixed otitis, there was no statistically significant difference (p > 0.05) between ear size (Table 16).

Table 16: Distribution of mixed otitis samples according to the size of the animal's ear.

Ear size	Mixed Insulation	%
Small	0	0
Average	7	43,7
Large	9	56,2
Total	16	100
(p > 0,05).		

4.20. Distribution of otitis samples according to the presence of ear hair:

Of the 36 animals, 17 (47.2%) had ear hair and 19 (52.8%) had no ear hair (graph 15). Most of the animals studied did not have hair on their ear tips.

Graph 15: Distribution of ear hair samples according to the presence of hair in the ears.

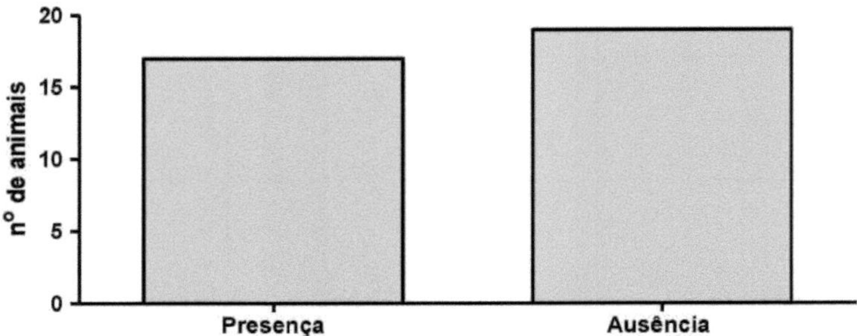

As for bacterial and non-bacterial otitis, there was a statistically significant difference ($p < 0.05$) between animals with or without inner ear hair (Table 17).

Table 17: Distribution of bacterial otitis samples according to the presence of ear hair.

Ear hair	Bacterial isolation	%
Hair on the ears	8	88,9
Absence of ear hair	1	11,1
Total	9	100
($p < 0,05$).		

As for fungal and non-fungal otitis, there was no statistically significant difference ($p > 0.05$) between animals with or without inner ear hair (Table 18).

Table 18: Distribution of fungal otitis samples according to the presence of ear hair.

Ear hair	Fungal isolation	%

Hair on the ears	5	55,5
Absence of ear hair	4	44,4
Total	9	100
(p > 0,05).		

With regard to mixed and non-mixed otitis, there was a statistically significant difference (p < 0.05) between animals with or without inner ear hair (Table 19).

Table 19: Distribution of mixed otitis samples according to the presence of ear hair.

Ear hair	Mixed Insulation	%
Presence of ear hair	3	18,7
No ear hair	13	81,2
Total	16	100
(p < 0,05).		

4.21. Distribution of ear secretion samples according to frequency of bathing:

Of the 36 animals, 14 (38.9%) were bathed weekly, six (16.7%) fortnightly, 12 (33.3%) monthly and four (11.1%) were not bathed (graph 16). Most of the animals that took part in the study were bathed weekly.

Graph 16: Distribution of ear secretion samples according to frequency of bathing.

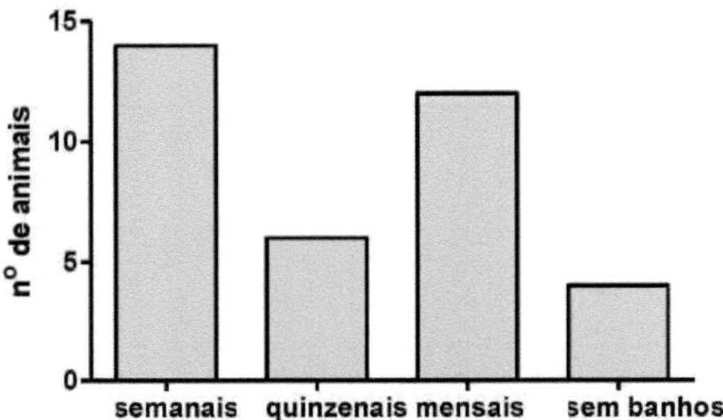

As for bacterial and non-bacterial otitis, there was no statistically significant difference (p > 0.05) when it came to bathing frequency (table 20).

Table 20: Distribution of bacterial otitis samples according to frequency of bathing.

Frequency of bathing	Bacterial isolation	%
Weekly Baths	5	55,5
Fortnightly baths	2	22,2
Monthly Baths	2	22,2
Not bathed	0	0
Total	9	100
(p > 0,05).		

As for fungal and non-fungal otitis, there was no statistically significant difference (p > 0.05) when it came to bathing frequency (table 21).

Table 21: Distribution of fungal otitis samples according to frequency of bathing.

Frequency of bathing	Fungal isolation	%
Weekly Baths	5	55,5
Fortnightly baths	1	11,1
Monthly Baths	3	33,3
Not bathed	0	0
Total	9	100
(p > 0,05).		

With regard to mixed and non-mixed otitis, there was a statistically significant difference (p < 0.05) when it came to bathing frequency (table 22).

Table 22: Distribution of mixed otitis samples according to frequency of bathing.

Frequency of bathing	Mixed Insulation	%
Weekly Baths	3	18,7
Fortnightly baths	3	18,7
Monthly Baths	6	37,5

Not bathed	4	25
Total	16	100
(p < 0,05).		

4.22. Distribution of otitis samples according to ear protection during bathing:

Of the 36 animals, nine (25%) received ear protection during their baths, while 27 (75%) did not (Graph 17). The largest proportion of animals in the study did not receive protection during their baths.

Graph 17: Distribution of samples regarding ear protection during baths.

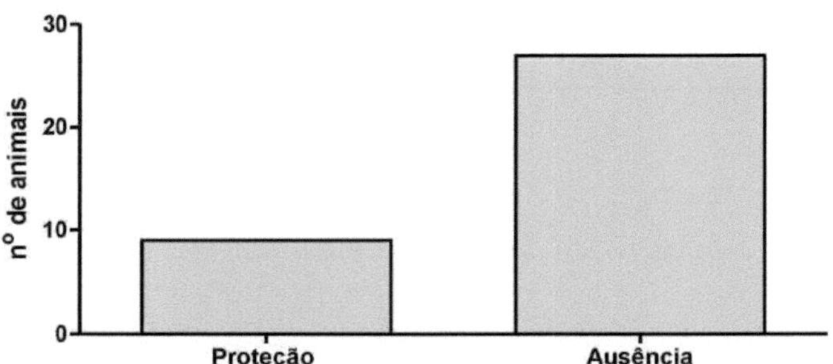

As for bacterial and non-bacterial otitis, there was no statistically significant difference ($p > 0.05$) in relation to the use of protection (table 23).

Table 23: Distribution of bacterial otitis samples according to ear protection.

Ear protection	Bacterial isolation	%

Protection	3	33,3
Absence	6	66,6
Total	9	100
(p < 0,05).		

As for fungal and non-fungal otitis, there was no statistically significant difference (p > 0.05) in relation to the use of protection (table 24).

Table 24: Distribution of fungal otitis samples according to the use of protection.

Ear protection	Fungal isolation	%
Protection	1	11,1
Absence	8	88,8
Total	9	100
(p < 0,05).		

As for mixed and non-mixed otitis, there was no statistically significant difference (ɔ > 0 05) in relation to the use of protection (table 25).

Table 25: Distribution of mixed otitis samples according to the use of protection.

Ear protection	Mixed Insulation	%
Protection	2	12,5
Absence	14	87,5
Total	16	100
(p < 0,05).		

4.23. Distribution of otitis samples in terms of ear hygiene:

Of the 36 animals, six (16.7%) performed ear hygiene and 30 (83.3%) did not (Graph 18). Most of the animals studied did not receive ear hygiene.

Graph 18: Distribution of ear secretion samples in terms of ear hygiene.

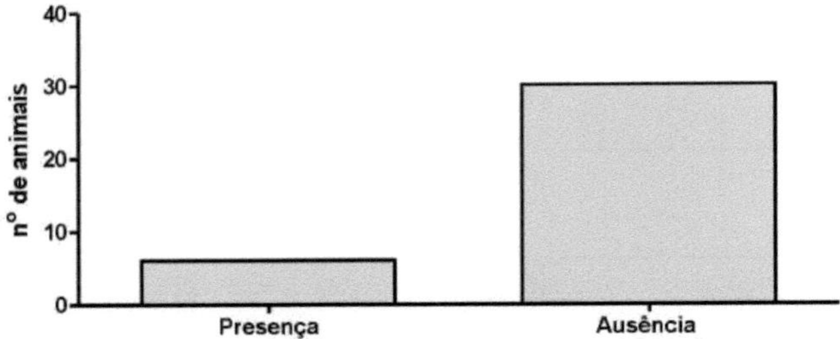

As for bacterial and non-bacterial otitis, there was no statistically significant difference (p > 0.05) in relation to ear hygiene practices (table 26).

Table 26: Distribution of bacterial otitis regarding the practice of ear hygiene.

Ear hygiene	Bacterial isolation	%
Presence	2	22,2

Absence	7	77,7
Total	9	100
(p < 0,05).		

With regard to fungal and non-fungal otitis, there was no statistically significant difference (p > 0.05) when it came to practicing ear hygiene (Table 27). None of the animals with mixed otitis received ear hygiene.

Table 27: Distribution of fungal otitis samples according to the practice of ear hygiene.

Ear hygiene	Fungal isolation	%
Presence	2	22,2
Absence	7	77,7
Total	9	100
(p < 0,05).		

4.24. Distribution of otitis samples according to contact with rain:

Of the 36 animals, 22 (61.1%) had contact with rain and 14 (38.9%) did not (Graph 19). The largest proportion of animals had contact with the rain.

Graph 19: Distribution of ear secretion samples according to exposure to rain.

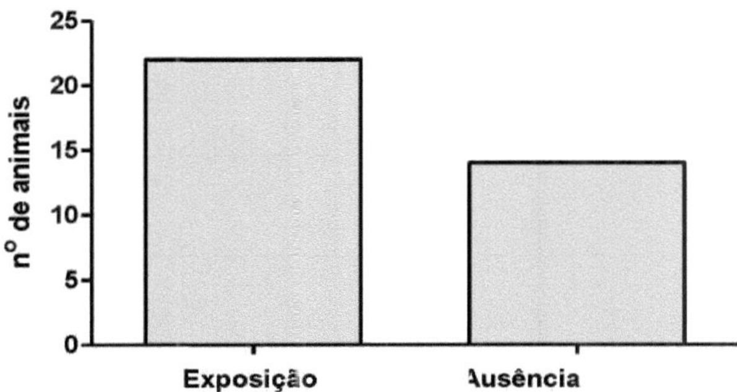

As for bacterial and non-bacterial otitis, there was no statistically significant difference (p > 0.05) in relation to exposure to rain (table 28).

Table 28: Distribution of bacterial otitis samples according to exposure to rain		
Exposure to rain	**Bacterial isolation**	**%**
Exhibition	5	55,5
Absence	4	44,4
Total	9	100
(p < 0,05).		

As for fungal and non-fungal otitis, there was no statistically significant difference ($p > 0.05$) in relation to exposure to rain (table 29).

Table 29: Distribution of fungal otitis samples according to exposure to rain		
Exposure to rain	**Fungal isolation**	**%**
Exhibition	6	66,6
Absence	3	33,3
Total	9	100
(p > 0,05).		

As for mixed and non-mixed otitis, there was no statistically significant difference ($p > 0.05$) in relation to exposure to rain (table 30).

Table 30: Distribution of mixed otitis samples according to exposure to rain		
Exposure to rain	**Mixed Insulation**	**%**
Exhibition	10	62,5
Absence	6	37,5
Total	16	100
(p < 0,05).		

4.25. Distribution of otitis samples according to the habit of frequenting aquatic environments:

Of the 36 animals, 23 (63.9%) had this habit and 13 (36.1%) did not (Graph 20). Most of the animals had the habit of frequenting the environment.

Graph 20: Distribution of ear secretion according to the habit of frequenting aquatic environments.

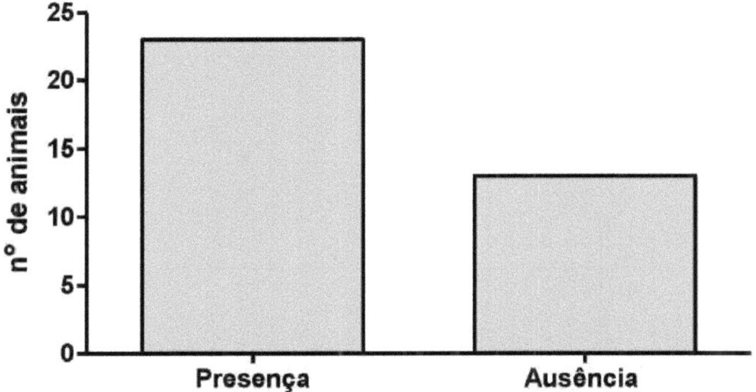

As for bacterial and non-bacterial otitis, there was no statistically significant difference (p > 0.05) in relation to the habit of frequenting aquatic environments (table 31).

Table 31: Distribution of bacterial otitis according to the habit of frequenting aquatic environments:

Contact with the aquatic environment	Bacterial isolation	%
Presence	7	77,7
Absence	2	22,2
Total	9	100
(p < 0,05).		

With regard to fungal and non-fungal otitis, there was no statistically significant difference (p > 0.05) when it came to the habit of frequenting environments (table 32).

Table 32: Distribution of fungal otitis according to the habit of frequenting aquatic environments.

Contact with the aquatic environment	Fungal isolation	%
Presence	7	77,7
Absence	2	22,2
Total	9	100
(p < 0,05).		

As for mixed and non-mixed otitis, there was no statistically significant difference (p > 0.05) in relation to the habit of frequenting environments (table 33).

Table 33: Distribution of mixed otitis according to the habit of frequenting aquatic environments:

Contact with the aquatic environment	Mixed Insulation	%
Presence	9	56,2
Absence	7	43,7
Total	16	100
(p < 0,05).		

4.26. Distribution of otitis samples according to residence:

Of the 36 animals, 31 (86.1%) lived in a yard and five (13.8%) lived in an apartment (Graph 21). Most of the animals lived in backyards.

Graph 21: Distribution of animals according to where they live:

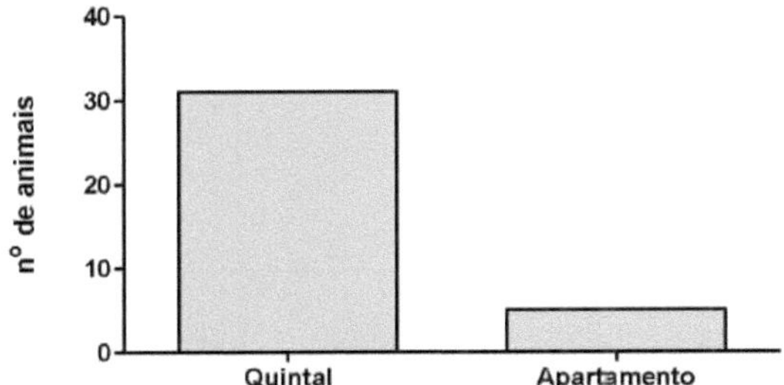

As for bacterial and non-bacterial otitis, there was no statistically significant difference (p > 0.05) in relation to housing (table 34).

Table 34: Distribution of bacterial otitis according to place of residence.

Housing	Bacterial isolation	%

Housing	Bacterial isolation	%
Backyard	7	77,7
Apartment	2	22,2
Total	9	100

(p < O,O5).

As for fungal and non-fungal otitis, there was no statistically significant difference (p > O,O5) in relation to housing (table 35).

Table 35: Distribution of fungal otitis according to place of residence.

Housing	Bacterial isolation	%
Backyard	8	88,8
Apartment	1	11,1
Total	9	100
(p < O,O5).		

As for mixed and non-mixed otitis, there was no statistically significant difference (p > 0.05) in relation to housing (table 36).

Housing	Mixed Insulation	%
Backyard	15	93,7
Apartment	1	6,2
Total	16	100

Table 36: Distribution of mixed otitis according to place of residence.

(p < 0,05).

4.27. Distribution of samples according to otitis classification:

5. Of the 36 animals, nine (25%) had bacterial otitis, nine (25%) fungal, 16 (44.4%) mixed and two (5.5%) aseptic (graph 22). A higher prevalence of mixed otitis was observed.

Graph 22: Distribution of samples according to otitis classification.

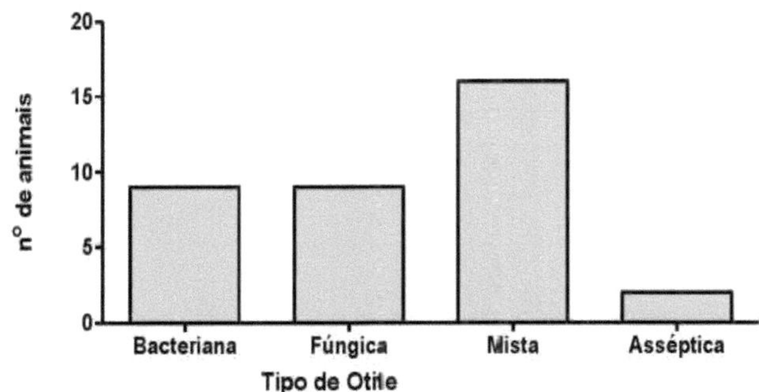

4.28. Distribution of samples according to the type of exudate:

Of the 36 animals, 16 (44.4%) had purulent exudate and 20 (55.6%) had ceruminous exudate (graph 23). Most of the animals studied had ceruminous exudate.

Graph 23: Distribution of samples according to the type of exudate:

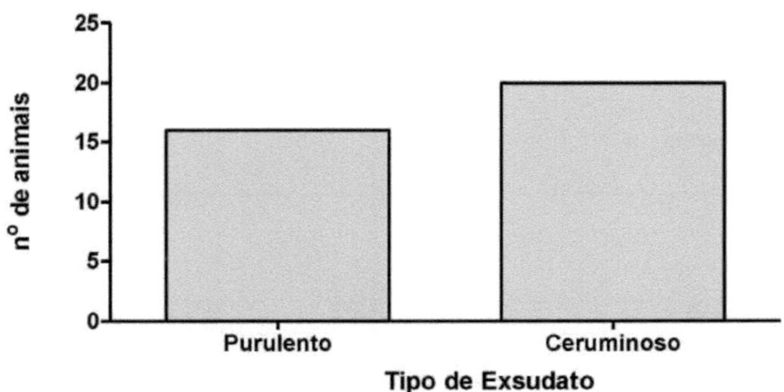

As for bacterial and non-bacterial otitis, there was a statistically significant difference (p < 0.05) in relation to the type of exudate (table 37).

Table 37: Distribution of bacterial otitis as to type of exudate.

Type of Exudate	Bacterial isolation	%
Purulent	9	100
Ceruminous	0	0
Total	9	100
(p < 0,05).		

As for fungal and non-fungal otitis, there was a statistically significant difference (p < 0.05) with regard to the type of exudate (table 38).

Table 38: Distribution of fungal otitis media according to the type of exudate.

Type of Exudate	Fungal isolation	%
Purulent	0	0
Ceruminous	9	100
Total	**9**	100

(p < 0,05).

As for mixed and non-mixed otitis, there was a statistically significant difference (p > 0.05) in relation to the type of exudate (table 39)

Table 39: Distribution of mixed otitis as to type of exudate.

Type of Exudate	Mixed Insulation	%
Purulent	7	75
Ceruminous	9	25
Total	**16**	100
(p < 0,05).		

4.29. Distribution of samples according to the type of otitis:

Of the 36 animals, four (11.1%) had acute otitis and 32 (88.9%) had chronic otitis (graph

24). Most of the animals studied had chronic otitis.

Graph 24: Distribution of animals according to the type of otitis.

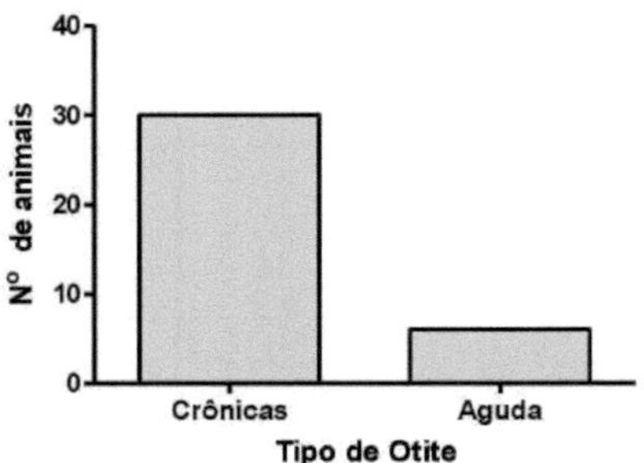

As for bacterial and non-bacterial otitis, there was no statistically significant difference (p > 0.05) in terms of type (table 40).

Table 40: Distribution of bacterial otitis by type.

Type of Otitis	Bacterial isolation	%
Chronicle	8	88,8
Acute	1	11,1
Total	9	100
(p < 0,05).		

As for fungal and non-fungal otitis, there was no statistically significant difference (p > 0.05) in terms of type (table 41).

Table 41 Distribution of fungal otitis by type.

Type of otitis	Fungal isolation	%

Chronicle	8	88,8
Acute	1	11,1
Total	9	100

(p < 0,05).

As for mixed and non-mixed otitis, there was no statistically significant difference (p > 0.05) in terms of type (table 42).

Table 42: Distribution of mixed otitis according to type.

Type of otitis	Mixed Insulation	%
Chronicle	16	100
Acute	0	0
Total	16	100

(p < 0,05).

4.30. Distribution of samples according to laterality:

Of the 36 animals, two (5.6%) had unilateral otitis, 34 (94.4%) bilateral (graph 25) . Most of the animals that took part in the study had bilateral otitis.

Graph 25: Distribution of animals according to otitis laterality.

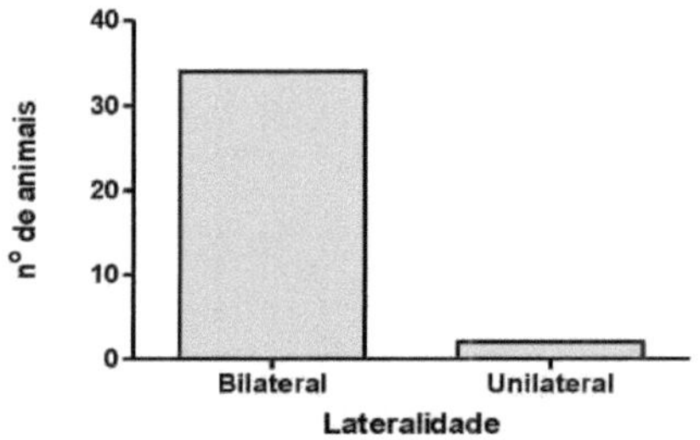

As for bacterial and non-bacterial otitis, there was no statistically significant difference (p > 0.05) in relation to laterality (table 43).

Table 43: Distribution of otitis as to laterality.

Laterality	Bacterial isolation	%
Unilateral	1	11,1
Bilateral	8	88,8
Total	**9**	100
(p < 0,05).		

As for fungal and non-fungal otitis, there was no statistically significant difference (p > 0.05) in relation to laterality (table 44).

Table 44: Distribution of otitis as to laterality.

Laterality	Fungal isolation	%
Unilateral	0	0
Bilateral	9	99,9
Total	**9**	100
(p < 0,05).		

As for mixed and non-mixed otitis, there was no statistically significant difference (p > 0.05) in relation to laterality (table 45).

Table 45: Distribution of otitis as to laterality.

Laterality	Mixed Insulation	%
Unilateral	1	6,2
Bilateral	15	93,7
Total	16	100

(p < 0,05).

4.31. Distribution of samples according to recurrence:

Of the 36 ears, 22 (61.1%) were recurrent and 14 (38.9%) were not (Graph 26). Most of the animals studied had recurrent otitis.

Graph 26: Distribution of animals with regard to relapses.

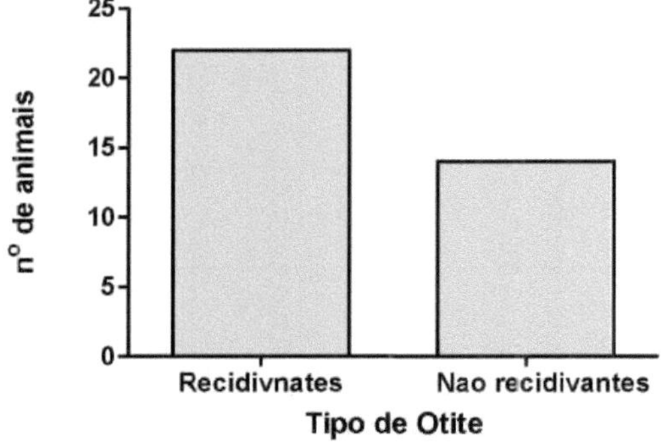

With regard to bacterial and non-bacterial otitis, there was a statistically significant difference (p < 0.05) when it came to recurrences.

Table 46: Distribution of otitis recurrences.		
Recurrences	Bacterial isolation	%
Recurring	7	77,7
Non-relapsing	2	22,2
Total	9	100
(p < 0,05).		

With regard to fungal and non-fungal otitis, there was no statistically significant difference (p > 0.05) when it came to recurrences, as well as mixed and non-mixed otitis.

Table 47: Distribution of fungal otitis recurrences.		
Recurrences	Fungal isolation	%
Recurring	3	33,3
Non-relapsing	6	66,6
Total	9	100
(p > 0,05).		

Table 48: Distribution of mixed otitis recurrences.		
Recurrences	Insulation Mixed	%
Recurring	12	75

Non-relapsing	4	25
Total	**16**	100
(p < 0,05).		

4.32. Distribution of samples in terms of pathological changes:

Of the 72 external ears examined, clinical inspection and otoscopic examination revealed that 30 (41.7%) had erythema, 48 (66.7%) had punctate hemorrhages, 54 (75%) had erosions, 62 (86.1%) had hyperemia, 52 (72.2%) had edema, 66 (91.7%) had thickened skin, 20 (27.8%) had hyperpigmentation, 28 (38.9%) had calcified cartilage, 52 (72,2%) periauricular abrasions, 22 (30.5%) partial stenosis, 19 (26.3%) brown exudate, 32 (44.4%) dark brown exudate, 24 (33.3%) yellow exudate, 50 (69.4%) intense exudate (50% or more of the otoscope cone obstructed), 20 (27.8%) moderate exudate (up to 50% of the otoscope cone obstructed), eight (11.1%) otohematoma. The prevalence of pathological changes observed was integumentary thickening followed by hyperemia.

4.33. Distribution of samples in terms of clinical alterations:

Of the 36 animals studied, 32 (88.9%) had pruritus, 36 (100%) had an altered odor, nine (25%) had hyperthermia, three (8.3%) had hypochlorous mucous membranes, three (8.3%) had mild dehydration, nine (25%) had inappetence, nine (25%) had an enlarged pre-parotid lymph node, five (13.9%) enlarged mandibular lymph nodes, 12 (33.3%) otalgia, five (13.9) altered ear position, 32 (88.9%) ear agitation and four (11.1%) head tilt. The highest prevalence observed was altered smell and itching.

4.34. Distribution of samples in terms of behavioral changes:

Of the 36 animals studied, 12 (33.3%) showed inattention, six (16.7%) depression, two (5.55%) aggression, two (5.55%) hearing loss, two (5.55%) excessive vocalization and one (2.8%) destroyed objects in the house (graph 27). The highest prevalence was observed in animals with inattention.

Graph 27- Behavioral changes in animals with otitis externa

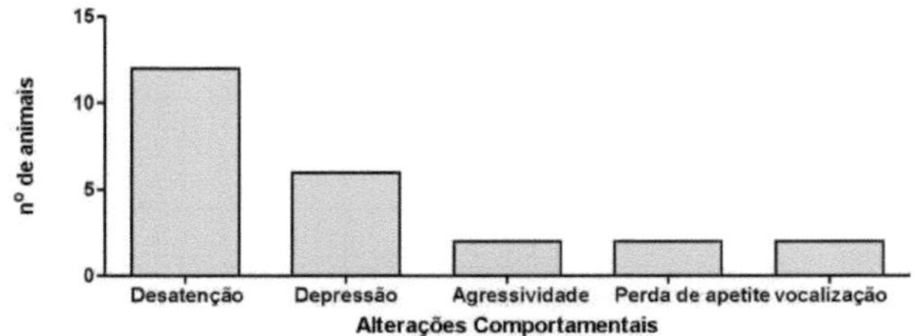

4.35. *In vitro* bacterial sensitivity patterns :

Table 49 shows the antimicrobials with regard to the *in vitro* bacterial sensitivity of 50 ear secretion samples. Resistance to at least one antimicrobial was observed in all the samples analyzed. The percentage of multiresistance (resistance to two or more antimicrobials) was 92%.

Table 49: Classification of antibiotics according to *in vitro* efficacy

Drugs	Sensitive	%	Intermediate	%	Resistant	%
Ampicillin	10	20	2	4	38	76
Amoxicillin	10	20	0	0	40	80
Amoxicillin acclav	19	38	0	0	31	62
Azithromycin	34	68	2	4	14	28
Bacitracin	4	8	0	0	46	92
Cephalothin	10	20	5	10	35	70
Cefoxitin	16	32	4	8	30	60
Ciprofloxacin	35	70	9	18	6	12
Clidamycin	30	60	3	6	17	34

Chloramphenicol	38	76	3	6	9	18
Enrofloxacin	37	74	1	2	12	24
Gentamicin	40	80	1	2	9	18
Neomycin	39	78	1	2	10	20
Penicillin	5	10	4	8	41	82
Polymyxin B	28	56	5	10	17	34
Sulfa c trimethoprim	14	28	2	4	34	68
Tetracycline	30	60	4	8	16	32
Tobramycin	36	72	2	4	12	24

4.36. List of antimicrobials with more than 70% *in vitro* efficacy:

Below are the percentages of *in vitro* sensitivity obtained by the antimicrobial agents that showed efficiency equal to or greater than 70% for the total group of samples: Chloramphenicol 76%, Ciprofloxacin 70%, Enrofloxacin 74%, Gentamicin 80%, Neomycin 78% and Tobramycin 72% (graph 28).

Graph 28: Distribution of samples *in terms* of *in vitro* sensitivity to the most effective antimicrobials:

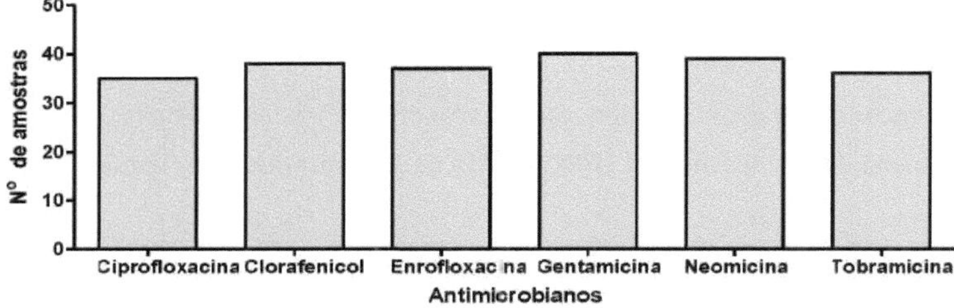

4.37. Intermediate response rate and *in vitro* sensitivity of antimicrobials with more than 70% efficacy from canine ear secretion samples:

Antibacterials, adding their intermediate response rates to *in vitro* sensitivity, in order to explain the potential of these drugs: Chloramphenicol - sensitivity (76%) and intermediate (6%) = 82%, Ciprofloxacin - sensitivity (70%) and intermediate (18%) = 88%, Enrofloxacin - sensitivity (74%) and intermediate (2%) = 76%, Gentamicin - sensitivity (80%) and intermediate (2%) = 82%, Neomycin - sensitivity (78%) and intermediate (2%) = 80%, Tobramycin - sensitivity (72%) and intermediate (4%) = 76%.

4.38. List of antimicrobials used in treatment and *in vivo* efficacy:

Of the 36 animals that took part in the study, 25 received treatment, nine with bacterial otitis and 16 with mixed otitis. Eight (32%) animals were treated with gentamicin, two of which were combined with oral enrofloxacin at a dose of 10 mg/kg every 24 hours for 12 days. Six (24%) were treated with topical neomycin. Six (24%) animals were treated with topical enrofloxacin. Five (20%) animals were treated with topical ciprofloxacin.

The clinical efficacy of gentamicin, neomycin and enrofloxacin was 100%.

The clinical efficacy of ciprofloxacin was 60%.

Of the 25 animals that received treatment, two had negative microbial isolation and unsatisfactory clinical improvement. The cure rate was 92%

4.39. Bacterial prevalence in ear secretion samples after treatment:

Four strains were isolated after treatment: *Pseudomonas sp* three (75%) and *Streptococcus sp* one (25%), corresponding to four samples of ear secretion.

All the animals that took part in the study had clinical signs of otitis, so the samples that were sterile (6.9%) can be explained by an error in collection, inadequate transportation, obtaining an ear sample during antimicrobial treatment or non-infectious otitis caused by allergic processes, mites, foreign bodies and contact with irritants (LOGAS, 1994, GRIFFIN, 1996, CURTIS, 2004). The negative samples in this study are considered low, an example of which is the percentage of 18.5% of negative cultures found by Lilenbaum et al (2000) in Rio de Janeiro, which was almost 3 times higher.

The observation of mixed infection (56.7%) was slightly higher than that obtained by Oliveira et al (2005), in Ceará, who obtained a frequency of 49.5% of polymicrobial infection. The high percentage of bacterial cultivation (76.4%) was even lower than that found by Oliveira et al (2005), who obtained 91.5%. The substantial bacterial isolation confirms the importance of bacterial causes in canine otitis.

Among the bacterial strains obtained, there was a greater number of gram-positive bacteria (56.4%), the most prevalent being the genus *Staphylococcus sp* 37.7%, including the species Staphylococcus *intermedius (19.9%), Staphylococcus* coagulase negative (9.9%) and *Staphylococcus aureus* (7.9%). The predominance of gram-positive bacteria was close to the 54% observed in Rio de Janeiro by Dieckmann et al (1996) and 55% obtained in the United States by Blue and Wooley (1977).

The predominance of *Staphylococcus sp* observed here confirmed previous studies carried out in dogs in Brazil, in the states of Pernambuco (Mota et al, 2000) and Mato Grosso do Sul (RIBEIRO et al., 2000), in Japan (YAMASHITA et al, 2005) and in France (ROUGIER et al., 2005), which found a prevalence of around 28, 25, 48 and 40 % for this genus respectively. On a specific level, the predominance of the *Staphylococcus intermedius* species in otopathic dogs in the present study confirmed previous results by Cole et al., 1998 and Lilenbaum et al., 2000.

In addition, this study found a high prevalence of *Pseudomonas sp from* ear samples of dogs with clinical signs of otitis externa, representing 26.7% of the bacteria isolated. Fernandez et al. (2006) also found a high prevalence of bacteria of this genus, with the most prevalent species being *Pseudomonas aeruginosa, isolated in* 22.2%, Cole et al. (1998) found isolates of *Pseudomonas aeruginosa* from the external ears (17.6%) and Petersen et al. (2002) found isolates of *Pseudomonas aeruginosa* in 27.8% of the samples analyzed. These percentages were close to those of bacteria of the same genus isolated in the present study. These authors suspect that this high incidence of *Pseudomonas aeruginosa* may be due to the increased virulence of this bacterium in tropical climates. The greater isolation of *Pseudomonas sp is* probably due to multiple bacterial infections, among which there was a high percentage of bacterial associations with the isolation of *Pseudomonas sp.* Oliveira et al. (2005), in Ceará, observed that the species *Pseudomonas aeruginosa,* the second most frequent bacterium, was more prevalent in mixed bacterial cultures than in single cultures, as was observed in the present study.

With regard to yeast isolation, 69.4% of the samples analyzed showed yeast growth, and the yeast *Malassezia pachydermatis* was found in all the cultures. Fernandez et al. (2006) isolated 69.3% of the *Malassezia pachydermatis yeast* and Crespo et al. (2000) found 68.4%, which is very close to the figure found in this study. Rougier et al. (2005) obtained 45% of positive mycological samples, with the yeast *Malassezia pachydermatis* isolated in 68.8%, a lower percentage than that found in this study. Nobre et al. (1998), Nobre et al. (2001) and Leite et al. (2003) found higher isolation rates for this yeast, 80.7%, 76.5% and 88% respectively. M. *pachydermatis is part of* the ear microbiota of domestic carnivores, although it can be pathogenic in different situations (Mansfield et al., 1990,

Leite et al., 2003). Samaneh et al., (2011) after investigating the different species of yeasts of the Malassezia genus on the skin and ear canal of healthy and sick dogs confirmed, as in this study, the presence of M. *pachydermatis* as the most prevalent in both groups. Mansifield et al. (1990) concluded after an experimental study with inoculation of *M. pachydermatis in* healthy dogs that this yeast is an opportunistic pathogen.

It was observed that 25% of otitis cases were caused exclusively by the yeast *Malassezia pachydermatis*. The percentage of cases of otitis caused exclusively by yeast (25%) found in this study was higher than that found in Sao Paulo by Larsson (1987), who found 15.1% of otitis due to mycotic causes, and the author included dogs and cats in his study. Meanwhile, Rougier et al. (2005), in France, found a lower figure than that found in this study, 8% of otitis caused by yeast. The possibility of otitis exclusively caused by yeast agents reinforces the need to send ear samples to both cultures in order to prescribe a more specific therapy (GRIFFIN,
1996), probably using a manipulated otologic solution containing only an antifungal ingredient. It is important to note that, although *Malassezia pachydermatis* is not the primary factor in yeast otitis, antifungal therapy should be instituted to remove the mycotic infection, in order to facilitate the investigation of the factor that is directly stimulating the occurrence of otitis (MORRIS, 1999).

The non-significant difference in the proportion of males and females in the animals that took part in this study, indicating no predilection of bacterial and mixed otitis in terms of the sex of the affected animals, confirmed the results of Dieckmann et al. (1996), but not Fernandez et al. (2006), who observed a higher proportion of affected females. However, a predilection in relation to sex was observed for mycotic otitis. The predominance of the age group between one and five years observed here confirmed the previous results of Fernadez et al. (2006) and Kiss et al. (1997). This result may have been due to the greater abundance of dogs studied in this age group.

Of all the animals that took part in the study, the most commonly observed dog breeds were the poodle and labrador retrivier breeds, as well as those with no defined breed. The profuse amount of hair inside the ear canal of poodle breed dogs has been reported as a predisposing factor to otitis (AUGUST, 1988). According to the survey carried out by Dieckmann et al. (1996), SRD animals were among the most affected animals, in agreement with this study. Oliveira et al. (2005) also found that poodle breed animals were the most common. Stout-Graham et al. (1990) concluded that dogs with a predisposition to otitis, such as labradors and cocker spaniels, even when healthy, have a greater number of apocrine glands than dogs of other breeds. These same authors observed that the number of apocrine glands is higher in dogs with otitis, suggesting a relationship between infection and the predominance of these glands.

In terms of physical attributes, most of the animals that took part in the study, i.e. all those with otitis, were medium or large in size, but when comparing the different types of otitis (bacterial, fungal or mixed) there was no statistically significant difference. Most of the animals had pendulous ears, but when bacterial and mixed otitis were compared there was no statistically significant difference. Ear morphology indicated a statistically significant difference in fungal otitis. Most of the animals that took part in the study had short coats; however, when compared to fungal otitis, there was no statistically significant difference. The type of coat indicated a statistically significant difference in bacterial and mixed otitis. Most of the animals had medium-sized and large ears, but when fungal and mixed otitis were compared there was no statistically significant difference. Ear size indicated a statistically significant difference for bacterial otitis. Most of the animals that took part in the study had ear hair, but when compared to fungal otitis there was no statistically significant difference. The presence of ear hair indicated a statistically significant difference in bacterial and mixed otitis media. According to Griffin et al., 1990 and Mansfield et al., 1990, large, pendulous-eared dogs are more affected, as seen in this study in relation to fungal otitis. Masuda et al. (2000) and Cafarchia et al. (2005) also observed that dogs with pendulous ears had more cases of otitis externa than those with erect ears. Hayes et al. (1997), in their study, found that dogs with upright ears, regardless of the amount of hair in the ear canals, had a lower prevalence of otitis. Huang and Huang (1999), when observing the temperature of the ear canal of normal dogs, found that ear canals with hair had lower temperatures than those without, suggesting that the temperature of the ear canal may be less important for the development of otitis externa, as found in this study. However, Logas, 1994, considers predisposing factors to be all the anatomical features that keep local humidity high and hinder ventilation of the ear canal, such as the shape of the ear (pendulous ear), excess hair inside the ear canal, as well as stenosed ear canals, as in Sharpei breed dogs. Yoshida et al. (2002), in a study similar to that of Huang and Huang (1999), measured the temperature and humidity of the external ear canal of healthy dogs and dogs with otitis and found no significant differences between these two groups of dogs. They suggested that the relative humidity of the ear canal does not predispose some breeds to developing otitis externa and also concluded that the type of ear (pendulous or erect) does not affect the retention of heat and humidity within the ear canal.

In terms of management practices, all of the animals with otitis received regular ear cleaning, but when comparing the different types of otitis (bacterial, fungal or mixed) there was no statistically significant difference. Excessive ear cleaning by owners can cause mechanical trauma to the ear canal and may be a predisposing factor to otitis (LOGAS, 1994; GRIFFIN, 1996). However, according to Rosychuk and Luttgen (2004), keeping the ear clean and dry is extremely important in controlling otitis externa. The accumulation of oily secretion, cerumen and *debris* can directly irritate the ear or contain microscopic foreign material that is irritating. *Debris* also produces a favorable microenvironment for the proliferation of bacteria and yeasts.

Of all the animals, the majority did not protect their ears during baths, were in contact with rain, and had a habit of frequenting aquatic environments; however, when the different types of otitis (bacterial, fungal or mixed) were compared, there was no statistically significant difference. Most of the animals studied were bathed weekly. In this study, the frequency of bathing indicated a statistically significant difference only with regard to mixed otitis. The habit of swimming, exposure to rain, and frequent bathing, especially when there is no mechanical blockage of water ingress, favor the ingress of water into the ear canal, altering the auricular microenvironment and increasing susceptibility to dermatological infections caused by bacteria and yeasts. Increased humidity inside the ear can influence the incidence of otitis externa in dogs, contributing to the growth of bacteria and fungi (YOSHIDA1, et al 2002). Moisture in the ear canal is therefore a key factor in *Malassezia pachydermatis* otitis, a fact confirmed by Mansfield et al. (1990) in the United States, who obtained positive cultures of *Malassezia pachydermatis* after daily inoculation of sterile saline solution into the ear canal of dogs for three weeks.

The higher number of animals that lived in the yard may be due to neglect because of the lesser proximity of the owner, who takes longer to notice the clinical signs of otitis. However, when comparing housing to the different types of otitis, there was no statistically significant difference.

Chronic and bilateral otitis predominated, but when comparing the evolution and laterality of the different types of otitis, there was no statistically significant difference. Farias et al., 2002 estimate that chronic otitis externa accounts for 76.7% of cases of otopathy in dogs, which was confirmed by this study. There was a higher prevalence of recurrent infections, with a statistically significant difference only for bacterial otitis. Irregular use and underdosing of otological products, especially when more than one active ingredient is combined, and without clinical and laboratory investigation, could lead to bacterial resistance and chronic and relapsing infections. The highest prevalence was also observed in animals with bilateral otitis, confirming the same conclusion made by Rose (1977).

According to Harvey et al. (2004), the presence of clinical signs and otoscopy, as seen in this study, are the main procedures for the clinical diagnosis of canine otitis externa. The most common pathological alteration observed was integumentary thickening followed by hyperemia. However, according to Fernandez et al (2006), itching and erythema of the external auditory canal are the most frequently observed otological signs in cases of otitis. The presence of stenosis was observed in many ears. In cases of chronic otitis externa, Harvey et al. (2004) stated that the epithelial lining of the external auditory canal reacts to inflammation with hyperplasia. Stenosis results from prolonged and constant inflammatory stimulation of the ear canal epithelium. The percentage of periauricular abrasions observed in this study was very close to that found by Oliveira et al (2006), who also found the occurrence of punctiform hemorrhages, erosions in the ear canal of dogs with associated otitis externa and otitis media and injuries to the pinna in higher percentages than those found in this study. Acute otological inflammations are characterized by erythema and swelling of the lining epithelium, so that the skin becomes easily traumatized and ulcerated and secondarily infected with the appearance of exudate. Most of the animals studied had a ceruminous exudate. When the type of exudate was compared to the different types of otitis, there was a significant difference. A high percentage of brown-colored exudate was observed. Adherent, serous and brown exudate is typical of staphylococcal or streptococcal infections and yellow exudate is characteristic of infections by gram-negative bacteria (ETINGER et al. 1992).

The highest prevalence observed was altered odor and itching. Bruyett and Lorenz (1993) mentioned, when discussing clinical aspects related to otitis externa and media, that the act of shaking the head and the visualization of trauma to the pinna are common signs of otitis externa, as was found in the present study. Oliveira et al (2006) found that otalgia and changes in the position of the ear were lower than those found in this study. Altered head position due to excessive pain may be a sign of associated otitis media.

With regard to behavioral changes, the most noticeable was the inattention of the animals affected by the disease. This disease is painful and causes extreme discomfort. Excessive pain can lead to the development of behavioral disorders such as aggression, excessive vocalization, isolation, inattention and depression. Negligence in the treatment and management of animals can lead to chronic and recurrent otitis externa, which can progress to otitis media with rupture of the tympanic membrane, resulting in loss of hearing and impairment of the vestibulo-cochlear apparatus, leading to disorientation and loss of quality of life.

In this study, the *in vitro* sensitivity obtained by the antimicrobial agents that showed efficiency equal to or greater than 70% for the total group of samples were: Chloramphenicol, Ciprofloxacin, Enrofloxacin, Gentamicin, Neomycin and Tobramycin. The classes of antimicrobials that showed *in vitro* sensitivity equal to or greater than 70% for the total group of samples were aminoglycosides (gentamicin, neomycin and tobramycin) and quinolones (ciprofloxacin and enrofloxacin). Gentamicin was the most sensitive antimicrobial *in vitro*.

One of the factors contributing to the high resistance to penicillin, ampicillin, amoxicillin, cephalothin and cefoxitin found in this study could be the production of B-lactamase by the S. intermedius strains, which is one of the bacteria with the highest percentage of isolations. When amoxicillin was combined with clavulanic acid, the percentage of sensitivity increased. This increase can be explained by the inhibition of the B-lactamase enzyme, amplifying the effects of the B-lactam antibiotic. A low rate of resistance to quinolones was observed in this study. However, the indiscriminate use of fluoroquinolones should be avoided, especially enrofloxacin, which could result in an increase in the resistance rate (JUNCO AND BARRASA, 2002). In this study, tobramycin and gentamicin indicated high sensitivity for the samples analyzed, in agreement with various studies (JUNCO E BARRASA, 2002, LEITE, 2003, OLIVEIRA,2005) which report high susceptibility rates against strains of *staphylococcus sp* isolated from canine otitis externa, the most prevalent genus in this study, and high efficacy in the topical treatment of this disease.

The clinical efficacy of gentamicin, neomycin and enrofloxacin was 100%. The clinical efficacy of ciprofloxacin was 60%. Four strains were isolated after treatment, *Pseudomonas sp* and *Streptococcus sp*, from four ear secretion samples corresponding to two animals with chronic and relapsing otitis.

Unlike yeast otitis, which does not require topical antibacterial agents, bacterial otitis requires simultaneous treatment with antibacterial and antifungal agents. This is justified because the changes in the microclimate of the ear canal caused by topical antibacterial therapy can predispose *Malassezia pachydermatis* to transform from commensal to pathogenic (MASON and EVANS, 1991).

After treatment, there was a reduction in pruritus, odor and erythema. It was observed that even in animals that did not have a negative microbial culture after treatment there was a reduction in clinical signs such as pruritus, unpleasant odor and exudate.

The cure rate was 92%. At the end of the treatment, 23 animals were cured and two had negative microbial isolation and unsatisfactory clinical improvement. The owners may have neglected the precepts of cleanliness, regular frequency of application and minimum duration of treatment, and failed to control or eliminate the factors involved in the process (predisposing, primary and perpetuating).

In this study, all the ear secretion samples analyzed were resistant *in vitro* to at least one of the antibiotics. The high percentage of multi-resistant samples found here may be a reflection of the high prevalence of canine otitis in the clinical care of companion animals and the excessive use of antibiotics without prior testing of the susceptibility profile, without the establishment of targeted and effective treatments. Bacterial resistance can be induced by the indiscriminate use of topical antimicrobials by dog owners, who often ignore the precepts of cleanliness, regular frequency of application and minimum duration of treatment. And the fact that the veterinarian resorts to culture and antibiograms when the patient already has a chronic condition or one that is difficult to resolve, a situation in which highly resistant bacteria have already been selected by previous therapies.

As such, this study reaffirms the need for individualized clinical assessment in cases of canine otitis externa and emphasizes the importance of microbial culture and antibiograms for the appropriate choice of antimicrobial to be adopted for effective treatment. However, it is clear that the success of otologic therapy will depend on controlling or eliminating the factors involved in the process (predisposing, primary and perpetuating), and failure to detect these will compromise the outcome of the treatment and may lead to chronicity and recurrences of the disease.

CONCLUSION

In canine otitis externa

- Bacteria of the genus *Staphylococcus sp.* were the most prevalent.

- Gram-positive bacteria predominated.

- The percentage of double bacterial cultures was higher than that of single and multiple bacterial cultures.

- The most common bacterial associations were *streptococcus sp* and *pseudomonas sp*, *pseudomonas sp, S. intermedins* and *E. coli.*

- The only yeast species isolated was *Malassezia pachydermatis.*

- Mixed cultures predominated.

- The most common association between bacteria and yeast was *Corynebacterium sp* and *M. pachydermatis.*

- The most frequent pathological alteration was integumentary thickening followed by hyperemia of the external auditory canal and altered odor followed by pruritus were the most common clinical alterations.

- Inattention was the most common behavioral alteration observed in the animals.

- Animals of the poodle breed predominated.

- There was no predilection for age.

- There was no predilection for bacterial otitis in relation to sex, size, ear morphology, frequency of bathing, exposure to rain, habit of frequenting aquatic environments, housing, protection and ear hygiene.

- Coat, ear size and the presence of ear hair influenced the presence of bacterial otitis.

- There was no predilection for fungal otitis in relation to size, coat, ear size, presence of hair in the ears, exposure to rain, the habit of frequenting aquatic environments, housing, frequency of bathing, protection and ear hygiene.

- Ear morphology influenced the presence of fungal otitis.

- There was no predilection for mixed otitis in relation to sex, size, ear size, exposure to rain, the habit of frequenting aquatic environments, housing or ear protection.

- The type of coat, the presence of hair in the ears and the frequency of bathing influenced the presence of mixed otitis.

- The origin of the otitis (bacterial, fungal or mixed) determines the type of exudate.

- The antibiogram testing 17 antimicrobials indicated a treatment efficiency of over 70% for Chloramphenicol, Ciprofloxacin, Enrofloxacin, Gentamicin, Neomycin or Tobramycin.

- The strains isolated after treatment were *Pseudomonas sp* and *Streptococcus sp.*

- The cure rate using gentamicin, neomycin, enrofloxacin and/or ciprofloxacin reached 92%.

- Gentamicin, neomycin and enrofloxacin showed better clinical efficiency in the treatment of canine otitis externa.

- The 21-day treatment ensured a reduction in clinical signs in all the animals.

BIBLIOGRAPHICAL REFERENCES

ANGUS, J.C.; LICHTENSTEIGER, C.; CAMPBELL, K.L.; SCHAEFFER, D.J. Breed variations in histopathologic features of chronic severe otitis externa in dogs: 80 cases (19952001). **Journal of American Veterinary Medical Association**. v. 221, n.7, p.1000-1006, 2002.

AUGUST, J.R. Otitis externa: a disease of multifactorial etiology. **Veterinary Clinic of North American Small Animal Practice**. n.18, p. 731-742, 1988.

BONATES, A. Otitis: detailed knowledge allows accurate diagnosis and successful treatment. **Vet. News**, v.62, p.6-8, 2003.

BLUE, J.L. WOOLEY, R.E. Antibacterial sensitivity patterns of bacteria isolated from dogs with otitis externa. **Journal of American Veterinary Medical Association**. v.171, n.4,p.362- 363, 1977.

BRUYETTE, D. S., LORENZ, M.D. Otitis externa and media: diagnostic and medial aspects. Sem. Small Anim., v. 8, p.3-9, 1993.

CAFARCHIA, C.; GALLO S.; CAPELLI G.; OTRANTO D. Occurrence and population size of *Malassezia* spp. in the external ear canal of dogs and cats both healthy and with otitis. **Mycopathology**. v.2, n.160, p.143-149, 2005.

COLE, L.K.; KWOCHKA, K.W.; KOWALSKI, J.J.; HILLIER, A. Microbial flora and antimicrobial susceptibility patterns of isolated pathogens from the horizontal ear canal and middle ear in dogs with otitis media. **Journal of the American Medical Association**. v.212, n.4, p.534-538, 1998.

CURTIS, C. F. Current trends in the treatment of *Sarcoptes*, *Cheyletiella* and *Otodectes* mites infestations in dogs and cats. **Veterinary Dermatology**. v.15, p. 108-114, 2004.

DIECKMANN, A. M.; TORRES, H.M.; FERREIRA, T.; AQUINO, M.H.C. Clinical aspects and antibacterial therapeutic evaluation of otitis externa in dogs. **Revista Brasileira de Medicina Veterinária**. v.18, n.6, p.242-245, 1996.

ETTINGER, S. J. Treatise on veterinary internal medicine. 3ed, v.4, Ed manole, 1992.

FARIAS, M.R. Otologic therapy. In: MANUAL DE TERAPÉUTICA VETERINÁRIA. 2.ed,. São Paulo: Editora Roca, 2002.

FERNANDEZ, G.; BARBOZA, G.; VILLALOBOS, A.; PARRA, O.; FINOL,G.; RAMIREZ, R.A. Isolation and identification of microorganisms present in 53 dogs suffering otitis externa. **Revista Científica**. v.16, n.1, p.23-30, 2006.

GRIFFIN, C. Cleaning and topical therapy of otitis. **Veterinary Hour**. n.94, p.17-25, 1996.

GIRAO, M.D.; PRADO, M.R.; BRILHANTE, R.S.; CORDEIRO, R.A.; MONTEIRO, A.J.; SIDRIM, J.J.; ROCHA, M.F. *Malassezia pachydermatis* isolated from normal and diseased external ear canals in dogs: A comparativeanalysis. **Veterinary Journal**. v.172, n.3, p.544548, 2005.

GINEL, P.J.; LUCENA, R.; RODRIGUEZ, J.C., ORTEGA, J. A semiquantitative cytological evaluation of normal and pathological samples from the external ear canal of dogs and cats. **J. Veterinary Dermatology**v.3, n.13, p. 151-156, 2002.

GOTTHELF, L.N. Factors that predispose the ear to otitis externa. In: GOTTHELF SMALL ANIMAL EAR DISEASES AN ILLUSTRATED GUIDE. 1.ed., p.16; 122, Philadelpnia: W.B. Saunders Company, 2000.

HAYES, H.M.; PICKLE, L.W.; WILSON, G.P. Effects of ear type and weather on the hospital prevalence of canine otitis externa. **Research in Veterinary Science**. v.3, n. 42, p. 294-298, 1987.

HEINE, P.A. Anatomy of the ear. In: Veterinary Clinics of North America Small Animal Practice Ear Disease. v.34, n.2, p. 379-395. Philadelphia: W.B. Saunders

Company. Guest editor Matousek, J.L.. March 2004.

KUMAR, A., ROMAN-AUERHAHN,M.R. Anatomy of the canine and feline ear. In: Gotthelf Small Animal Ear Diseases an Illystrsted. Guide. 1.ed., p.1-23. Philadelpria: W.B. Saunders Company, 2000.

HUANG, H.P.; HUANG, H.M. Effects of ear type, sex, age, body weight, and climate on temperatures in the external acoustic meatus of dogs. American **Journal of Veterinary Research.** v. 9, n.60, p.1173-1176, 1999.

JACOBSON, L.S. Diagnosis and medical treatment of otitis externa in the dog and cat. JOURNAL OF THE SOUTH AFRICAN VETERINARY ASSOCIATION. v.4, n.73, p.162170, 2002.

KISS, G.; RADVANYI, S.; SZIGETI, G. New combination for the therapy of canine otitis externa. I. Microbiology of otitis externa. **Journal of Small Animal Practice.** v.38, n.2, p.5156, 1997.

LARSSON, C. E. **Contribution to the study of otopathies in dogs and cats.** Sao Paulo, 1987. 182 f. Thesis (Post Doctorate). Faculty of Veterinary Medicine and Zootechny, University of Sao Paulo.

LEITE, C.A.L Otitis in dogs and cats. In: EPIDEMIOLOGIA. CAES GATOS, v.15, p.2226, 2000.

LEITE, C.A.L; ABREU, V.L.V.; COSTA, G.M. Frequency of *Malasseziapachydermatis* in otitis externa of dogs. **Arquivo Brasileiro de Veterinaria e Zootecnia.** v.55, n.1, p. 101-104, 2003.

LEITE, C.A.L. Topical and systemic therapies: skin, ear and eye. In: MANUAL DE TERAPÊUTICA VETERINÁRIA. 3.ed., p.168-179, Sao Paulo: Editora Roca, 2008.

LILENBAUM, W., VERA, M.; SOUZA, G.N. Antimicrobial susceptibility of staphylococci isolated from otitis externa in dogs. **Letters in Applied Microbiology,** 31, p. 42-45, 2000.

LOGAS, D.B. Diseases of the ear canal. **Veterinary Clinic of North American Small Animal Practice.** v.5, n.24, p. 905, 1994.

MASON, K.V.; EVANS, A.G. Dermatitis associated with *Malasseziapachydermatisin* 11 dogs. **Journal of the American Animal Hospital Association.** v. 27, p.13-20, 1991.

MANSFIELD, P.D.; BOOSSINGER, T.R.; ATTLELERGER, M.H. Infectivity of *Mallassezia pachydermatisin* the external ear canal of dogs. **Journal of the American Animal Hospital Association.** v.26, p.97-100, 1990.

MASUDA, A.; SUKEGAWA, T.; MIZUMOTO, N.; TANI, H.; MIYAMOTO, T.; SASAI, K.; BABA, E. Study of lipid in the ear canal in canine otitis externa with *Malassezia pachydermatis*. **Journal of Veterinary Medical Science.** v. 11, n. 62, p. 1177-1182, 2000.

MOTA, R.A.; FARIAS, J.K.O.; SILVA, L.B.G.; LIMA, E.T.; OLIVEIRA, A.A.F.; MOURA, R.T.D. Efficacy of Otomax in the treatment of bacterial and fungal otitis in dogs. **Hora Veterinária.** v. 19, n., p. 13-16, 2000.

MORRIS, D.O. *Malassezia* dermatitis and otitis. **Veterinary Clinic of North American Small Animal Practice.** v.6, n.29, p.1303-1310, 1999.

NOBRE, M.O.; MEIRELES, M.C.A.; GASPAR, L.F.; PEREIRA, D.; SCHRAMM, R.; SCHUCH, L.F.; SOUZA, L.; SOUZA, L. *Malassezia pachydermatis* and other infectious agents in otitis externa and dermatitis in dogs. **Ciência Rural.** v.28, n.3, p.447-452, 1998.

NOBRE, M.O.; CASTRO, A.P.; NASCENTE, P.S.; FERREIRO, L.; MEIRELES, M.C. Occurrence of *Malassezia pachydermatis* and other infectious agents as a cause of otitis externa in dogs in the State of Rio Grande do Sul, BR (1996/1997). **Brazilian Journal of Microbiology.** v.32, n.3, p.245-249, 2001.

OLIVEIRA, L.C.; MEDEIROS, C.M.O.; SILVA, I.N.G.; MONTEIRO, A.J.; LEITE, C.A.L.; CARVALHO, C.B.M. Susceptibility to antimicrobials of bacteria isolated from otitis externa in dogs. **Arquivo Brasileiro de Medicina Veterinária e Zootecnia.** v.57, n.3, p.405-408, 2005.

OLIVEIRA, L.C.; BRILHANTE, R.S.N., CUNHA, A.M.S.; CARVALHO, C.B.M. Profile of microbial isolation in dogs with associated otitis media and external otitis. **Arquivo Brasileiro de Medicina Veterinária e Zootecnia.** v.58, n.6, p.1009-1017, 2006.

PETERSEN, A.D.; WALKER, R.D.; BOWMAN, M.M.; SCHOTT, H.C.; ROSSER, E.J. Jr. Frequency of isolation and antimicrobial susceptibility of Staphylococcus intermedius and Pseudomonas aeruginosa isolates from canine skin and ear samples over a 6-year period (1992-1997). **Journal of the American Animal Hospital Association.** v.38, p.407-413, 2002.

QUINN, P.J.; MARKEY, B.K.; CARTER, M.E.; DONNELLY, W.J.; LEONARD, F.C. MICROBIOLOGIA VETERINARIA E DOENCAS INFECCIOSAS.Porto Alegre, Brazil: Artmed, 2005.

RIBEIRO, L.R.R.; GONFIANTINI, J.M.P.F.; BABO, V.J.; BASTOS, O.P. Flora bacteriana de ouvido de caes atendidos no hospital veterinário da UFMS. **Hora Veterinária.** n.118, p.29-31, 2000.

ROUGIER, S.; BORELL, D.; PHEULPIN, S.; WOEHRLE, F.; BOISRAME, B. A comparative study of two antimicrobial/anti-inflammatory formulations in the treatment of canine otitis externa.**Veterinary Dermatologyv.**5, n.16, p.299-307, 2005.

ROSE, WR. Small animal clinical otology. Surgery 1--myringotomy. Number twenty-two in a series. **Veterinary Medicine and small Animal Clinician.** v.10, n.72, p.1646-1650, 1977.

ROSSER, E. J. Jr. Causes of otitis externa. In: VETERINARY CLINICS OF NORTH AMERICA SMALL ANIMAL PRACTICE EAR DISEASE. v.34, n.2, p.459. Philadelphia:
Publisher W.B. Saunders Company. Guest editor Matousek, J.L.. March 2004.

ROSYCHUK and LUTTGEN, Eyes, ears, nose and throat. In: TRATADO DE MEDICINA INTERNA VETERINARIA DOENQAS DO CAO E DO CATO. 5.ed., p. 10481056, Rio de Janeiro: Editora Guanabara Koogan, 2004.

SCOTT, D.W.; MILLER, W.H.; GRIFFIN, C.E. Diseases of eyelids, claws, anal sacs, and ears. In: MULLER & KIRK'S SMALL ANIMAL DERMATOLOGY. 6.ed., p.1204-1231, Philadelpnia: W.B. Saunders Company, 2001.

TANER, K. C., SCOTT, D. W., MILLAR, W. H., ERB, H. N.. The Cytology of the External Ear Canal in the Normal Dog and Cat, J. Vet. Med. A 50, p. 370-374, 2003.

TATER, K.C.; SCOTT, D.W.; MILLER Jr, W.H.; ERB, H.N. The cytology of the external ear canal in the normal dog and cat. **Journal of Veterinary Medicine.** v.50, p. 370-374, 2003.

YOSHIDA, N., NAITO1, F., FUKATA1, T., Studies of Certain Factors Affecting the Microenvironment and Microflora of the External Ear of the Dog in Health and Disease, *J. Vet. Med. Sci.* p. 1145-1147, 2002.

YAMASHITA, K.;SHIMIZU, A.; KAWANO, J.; UCHIDA, E.; HARUNA, A.; IGIMI, S. Isolation and characterization of Staphylococci from externa auditory meatus of dogs with or without otitis externa with special reference to *Staphylococcus schleiferi* sub sp. *coagulans* isolates. **Journal of Veterinary MedicineScience.**v.67, n.3, p.263-268, 2005.

GINEL, P. J., LUCENA, R., RODRIGUEZ, J. C., ORTEGA, J.,A semi quantitative cytological evaluation of normal and pathological samples from the external ear canal of dogs and cats,*Veterinary Dermatology*, vol. 13, p. 151-156, 2002.

STOUT-GRAHAM, M.; KAINER, R.A.; WHALEN, R.; MACY, D.W. Morphologic measurements of the external horizontal ear canal of dogs. **Journal of VeterinaryResearch.** v.51, n.7, p.990-994, 1990.

WHITE, R.A.S.; POMEROY, C.J. Total ear cana ablation and lateral bulla osteotomy in the dog. **Journal of Small Animal Practice.** 31, p.547-553, 1990.

CRESPO, M.J., ABARCA, M.L., CABANES, M.L., Atypical lipid-dependent *Malassezia* species isolated from dogs whit otitis externa. **J. Clin. Microbiol.**, v.38, p.2383-2385, 2000.

HARVEY, R.G., HARARI, J., DELAUCHE, A.J. **Ear** diseases in **dogs and cats.** Rio de Janeiro, Editora Revinter, 2004. 272p.

JUNCO, M.T.T., BARRASA, J.T.M. Indentification and antimicrobial susceptibility of coagulase positive Staphylococci isolated from healthy and dogs suffering from otitis externa. **Journal of Brazilian Veterinary Medicine**, v. 49, p. 419-423, 2002.

Samaneh EID, Ali Reza KHOSRAV, Shahram JAMSHID, A comparison of different kinds of Malassezia species in healthy dogs and dogs with otitis externa and skin lesions. Turk. J.
Vet. Anim. Sci. 2011; 35(1): doi:10.3906/vet-1007-412, 2011.

MANISCALCO, C.L., AQUINO, J.O., PASSOS, R.F.B., BURGER., C.P., MORAES., P.A., Use of video-otoscopy in the diagnosis of otitis externa in dogs. **Ciencia Rural, Santa Maria,** v.39., n.8., p.2454-2457, 2009.

Malayeri H.Z., Jamshidi, S., Salehi, T.Z., Identification and antimicrobial susceptibility patterns of bacteria causing otitis externa in dogs. **Vet Res Commun** 34:435-444, 2010.

Penna, B., Varges, R., Medeiros, L., Martins, G.M., Martins, R.R., Lilenbaum, W. Species distribution and antimicrobial susceptibility of staphylococci isolated from canine otitis externa. **Veteniray dermatology** DOI: 10.1111/j.1365-3164.2009.00842., 2009.

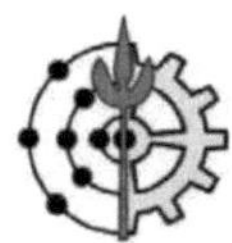

FEDERAL RURAL UNIVERSITY OF RIO DE JANEIRO
POSTGRADUATE COURSE IN VETERINARY MEDICINE
PATHOLOGY AND CLINICAL SCIENCES

CLINICAL FILE

Name: Raga: Age: Sex: ( ) M ( ) F Coat: ( ) Short ( ) Long Size: ( ) P ( )M ( ) G ( ) GG Ear type: ( ) Pendular
( ) Semi-Pendular ( ) Erect ( ) G   ( ) P
Ear hair: ( ) Yes ( ) No

Clinical Parameters:
Rectal temperature:Lymph nodes:Mucosal staining:
Behavioral Changes:Skin turgor: Appetite: _________________________ Stool:
Concomitant illness: ____
Use of medication: ____

Clinical examination of the external auditory canal:
Right ear canal (1) Left ear canal (2)
( ) Erythema ( ) Hyperemia ( ) Itching ( ) Hyperpigmentation ( ) Crust ( ) Exudate Color: ( )   Pain
sensitivity ( ) Unpleasant odor
( ) Duct thickening ( ) Auricular cartilage calcification ( ) Cerumen enlargement Color: ( )   Head tilt
( ) Ear agitation   ( ) Periauricular excoriation   ( ) Edema
Complementary observations of otoscopy: ____

Otitis Externa
( ) Unilateral ( ) Bilateral ( ) Acute ( ) Chronic ( ) Relapsing
( ) Purulent ( ) Ceruminous

Management
Frequency of bathing: ( ) Weekly ( )   Monthly ( ) Fortnightly ( ) No bathing
Protect your ear with cotton wool: ( ) Yes ( ) No
Ear hygiene: ( ) Yes ( ) No ( ) Ear solution ( ) Cotton only Frequency:
Ear hair removal: ( ) Yes ( ) No
Does it get rained on: ( ) Yes ( ) No
Enters: ( ) Lakes ( ) Sea ( ) River ( ) Swimming pool ( )No
Dwelling: ( ) Apartment   ( ) House( ) Farm ( ) Backyard
Other animals: ( ) Yes   ( ) NoSpecies/how many ____________ :
Ectoparasites: ( ) Flea ( ) Tick   ( ) Louse
Date: /   /Owner: ____________________

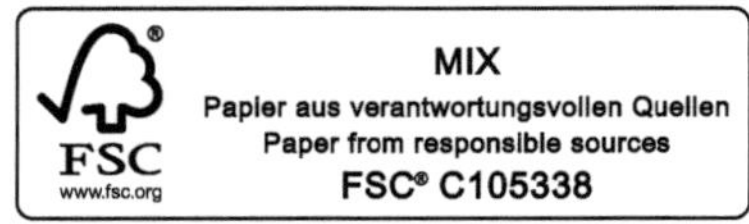

Printed by Books on Demand GmbH, Norderstedt / Germany